Personality Disorders Over Time

Precursors, Course, and Outcome

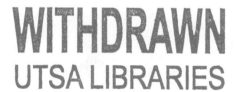

Personality Disorders Over Time

Precursors, Course, and Outcome

Joel Paris, M.D.

Professor of Psychiatry
McGill University
Montreal, Quebec, Canada

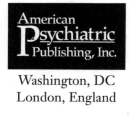

Washington, DC
London, England

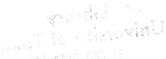

Copyright © 2003 American Psychiatric Publishing, Inc.
ALL RIGHTS RESERVED

Manufactured in the United States of America on acid-free paper
07 06 05 04 03   5 4 3 2 1
First Edition

Typeset in Adobe's Janson Text and ChapaMM

American Psychiatric Publishing, Inc.
1000 Wilson Boulevard
Arlington, VA 22209-3901
www.appi.org

Library of Congress Cataloging-in-Publication Data
Paris, Joel, 1940–
    Personality disorders over time : precursors, course, and outcome / Joel Paris.
        p. cm.
    Includes bibliographical references and index.
    ISBN 1-58562-040-8 (alk.paper)
    1. Personality disorders--Longitudinal studies. 2. Personality disorders--Treatment. I. Title.

    RC554.P369 2003
    616.85′8--dc21

                                                                    2002043871

British Library Cataloguing in Publication Data
A CIP record is available from the British Library.

This book is dedicated to my daughters, Leslie and Nancy, who give me continuity over time.

Contents

Introduction

Why Personality Disorders Are Important

All therapists treat patients with personality disorders. Some do so by choice, others by chance. Personality change has long been the central goal of extended courses of treatment. Clinicians whose practices center on long-term psychotherapy are interested in patients with personality disorders. These therapists are not satisfied with only relieving immediate distress but aim for more, seeking to modify personality.

Patients with personality disorders are difficult. Many clinicians attempt, whenever possible, to *avoid* treating them (Lewis and Appleby 1988). Yet even practitioners with no special interest in personality disorders are forced to grapple with the problem. In practice, most therapy focuses on managing symptoms. We administer courses of therapy that are effective for most patients, yet we find ourselves spending more time on the significant minority that fails to respond. Many of these "treatment-resistant" patients meet diagnostic criteria for personality disorders, and as I show in this book, approaches that are effective for Axis I disorders can sometimes be counterproductive for Axis II pathology.

Clinicians sometimes acknowledge this problem by describing difficult patients as having "Axis II comorbidity." This way of thinking implies that Axis I symptoms such as depression or anxiety are the main issue, albeit complicated by Axis II pathology. Yet in many cases, it would make more sense to make a primary diagnosis of personality disorder and then to speak of "Axis I comorbidity."

Patients with personality disorders have chronic problems in many areas of their lives, making them less than popular with clinicians. This book is *about* chronicity. To understand disorders with a chronic course, we must know how they evolve over time. The precursors, the onset, and the outcome of personality disorders constitute a meaningful sequence shedding light on their origins. Moreover, their course over time suggests a practical approach to therapy.

Why Clinicians Avoid Diagnosing Personality Disorders

I have long been puzzled by the reluctance of clinicians to diagnose personality disorders. Since 1972, I have been supervising psychiatric residents in a clinic that provides about 300 consultations a year to the community. We routinely make Axis II diagnoses, carefully following the criteria spelled out in the *Diagnostic and Statistical Manual of Mental Disorders* (DSM). I try to avoid overdiagnosing these conditions simply because of my special interest. All the same, when the patients referred to me have chronic problems in work and relationships, a personality disorder may be my primary diagnosis. In these cases, no other construct accounts for such a broad range of difficulties over so long a time.

Some clinicians believe that it is difficult to diagnose a personality disorder in one interview. Yet, with experience, I can usually obtain a personal history detailed enough to identify Axis II pathology with some accuracy. When I cannot obtain enough data, the patient has probably not told me the whole story. Because personality pathology can be ego-syntonic, I may need an informant to describe relationship patterns. In these cases, I ask the patient to return for a second interview, accompanied by a family member.

Early diagnosis of a personality disorder has a great clinical advantage. If you know this much about a patient, you will not be surprised when he or she presents treatment difficulties or fails to respond to methods that are effective for others. You can also adjust your expectations to chronicity. Unfortunately, many patients, even those who clearly meet the diagnostic criteria for a personality disorder, receive not Axis II diagnoses but multiple Axis I diagnoses.

This reluctance to make an Axis II diagnosis is only partly irrational. There are serious problems with the validity of the current categories of personality disorder (Nurnberg et al. 1994). Many years ago, Heinz Lehmann, one of my most esteemed teachers and a world-recognized expert on psychopathology, advised me to avoid using the term *borderline personality* because "nobody knows what it means." At that time, Heinz was probably right. Since then, however, great progress has been made in defining the category. All the same, major problems remain for the validity of all the Axis II diagnoses—not to speak of the fuzzy boundary between traits and disorders.

Yet, to put the issue in perspective, the situation for Axis I disorders is not much better. We do not really know the precise boundaries of schizophrenia. We have been unable to determine if it is one disease or many, or how to separate it clearly from other psychoses (Siever et al. 1993). Even constructs as basic to practice as depression and anxiety have ambiguous boundaries with other disorders—as well as with normality (Goldberg 2000). Many currently fashionable categories, such as posttraumatic stress disorder, have problems with diagnostic validity (Bowman 1999).

The creation in the DSM system of a special axis for personality traits and disorders was a serious attempt to focus the attention of clinicians. Ironically, it has succeeded only in creating an "Axis II ghetto," in which personality disorders are isolated and ignored. Some think it would be more helpful to diagnose personality disorders on Axis I, leaving trait profiles on Axis II (Livesley, in press). For busy clinicians, five axes can be four too many. In practice, most attention goes into establishing an Axis I diagnosis. When I read written reports that list all five axes, they tend to hedge—with descriptors such as "Axis II: deferred" or "Axis II: borderline traits."

The main resistance to diagnosing personality disorders, however, arises from their very nature. DSM-IV-TR (American Psychiatric Association 2000) describes these conditions as *stable* patterns that can be *traced back* to adolescence or early childhood, leading to *long-term* difficulties that seriously interfere with the capacity for work and/or stable relationships. Thus, by definition, these diagnoses describe *chronic* difficulties that can endure for a lifetime. Is it any wonder that some clinicians prefer not to think in these terms about their patients? Is it not more gratifying to focus on a recent episode of depression, which one can expect to treat successfully?

In my experience, patients tend to earn a personality disorder diagnosis only at the point when their treatment has failed. It is no fantasy that this population tends not to do well in therapy. For example, those who have an Axis I mood disorder and who *also* meet criteria for an Axis II diagnosis tend to respond more poorly to both psychological and pharmacological interventions (Shea et al. 1990). Personality pathology itself changes slowly at best. This is the case even for the best researched and most effective modes of treatment (Gunderson 2001; Linehan 1993; Livesley, in press).

The rule for personality disorders seems to be "out of sight, out of mind." Yet these conditions are very common. Their exact community prevalence depends on where one draws the boundary between traits and disorders. Most estimates range above 10% (Casey 2000; Weissman 1993), but because it is difficult to determine whether psychopathology is clinically significant (Narrow et al. 2002), this figure may be too high. Yet even if we were to halve that estimate, an enormous number of people could have personality disorders.

We have more precise information about the prevalence of antisocial personality disorder, which has been shown repeatedly to affect at least 2%

of the population, twice as many as suffer from either schizophrenia or bipolar illness (Kessler et al. 1994; Newman and Bland 1998). Judging from the most recent community surveys (Samuels et al. 2002; Torgersen et al. 2001), the prevalence of borderline personality disorder (BPD) is lower than that. BPD cases *seem* more common because patients with BPD are highly treatment-seeking. The forthcoming National Comorbidity Replication, to be led by Ronald Kessler, will be the first epidemiological survey in North America to specifically examine the community prevalence of BPD and will provide more precise data.

Personality disorders may be more common in the clinic than in the community. A recent study (Gross et al. 2002) found that patients with BPD make up 6% of all those seen in primary care. About 25% of patients attending psychiatric clinics, whatever other diagnoses they have, also have Axis II disorders (Casey 2000; Lewis and Appleby 1988). When we avoid diagnosing personality disorders, this leads to serious failure in assessing one-quarter of our patients.

How I Became a Researcher in Personality Disorders

My own interest in personality disorders goes back to the time of my training, over 30 years ago. In the heyday of psychodynamic psychiatry, personality disorders were believed to be definitively treatable, the most common prescription being long-term intensive psychotherapy. Although no documentation for the effectiveness of this method existed, we were not yet living in the era of "evidence-based practice." By and large, we took what our teachers told us on faith. Because nobody could know how long therapy might last, we never actually saw the marvelous results we heard or read about. But we *believed*.

In retrospect, our education was based on theories of the origins of personality disorder that we now know to be wrong. It is no longer tenable to claim that the causes of personality pathology lie mainly in early experiences; the relationship between childhood experiences and adult outcomes is too complex to support that conclusion (Paris 2000c; Rutter 1989). Moreover, unearthing and interpreting childhood experiences is not necessarily the most effective way to treat patients with personality disorders. Some therapists are still attracted by the receding mirage of "mutative" interventions—that is, precise and sweeping interpretations that are purported to lead to dramatic changes (Malan 1979). Yet, as this book shows, we lack firm evidence that patients with personality disorders consistently respond to long-term intensive therapy. The method might be best reserved for a selected minority of patients, such as those who, in spite of their difficulties, function at a higher level (Paris 1998b).

Although it misled us with simplistic conclusions, the heady atmosphere of the 1960s had a good side. Psychiatry residents were interested in personality and in understanding mental structures. We were actually *eager* to make personality disorder diagnoses, as a way of accounting for the fascinating inner world of our patients. Today, mental health professionals are most interested in symptom relief, and the grandiose goals of the past have been dismissed in favor of a hard-headed practicality. In psychiatry, the biomedical model has been steadily marginalizing training in psychotherapy (Luhrmann 2000). Patients with personality disorders are accordingly of less interest, and fewer are offered extensive courses of treatment.

Yet lack of interest has not made these patients disappear. Many move in and out of the mental health system; they turn up in a crisis and then are not seen again until the next time they get into trouble. The more seriously disturbed patients, such as those with BPD, are more likely to remain in clinical settings. As clinicians know, these patients make difficult demands and are not known for being grateful for what therapists have to offer.

Patients who are this problematic can receive labels reflecting therapist frustration. The term *treatment-resistant depression* (Trivedi and Kleiber 2001) shamelessly begs the question as to *why* such these patients' depression fails to respond to methods that work for others. I suggest in this book that many patients with personality disorders are overmedicated. For example, it is not unusual for patients with BPD to be taking four or five drugs, none of which controls their symptoms (Zanarini et al. 2001). I intend to show that although therapy with these patients is difficult, we have better evidence for its effectiveness than we do for pharmacological interventions.

Clinicians, like everyone else, yearn for success, but personality disorder cases are tainted with failure. These patients become the ones clinicians love to hate. Once the diagnosis is made, professionals run in the other direction. Another common response is to ignore chronicity, dismiss previous failures, and rediagnose the patient's disorder in line with the latest and trendiest theories.

This book aims to refute all these attitudes. Treatment of personality disorders must begin, at the very least, with recognition of their chronic course. Instead of ignoring chronicity, we must find out what it is telling us.

Long-Term Outcome: A Personal Narrative

All lives are narratives. Each has a beginning, a middle, and an end. Illnesses also have unique stories, characterized by precursors, course, and outcome.

My own interest in the subject also has its story. I have always been interested in outcome. Even as a child, I felt that narratives ended too soon. When I expressed frustration at not knowing what happened to the characters in some television drama, my father would tease me: "Do you really need to know their whole life?" Yes, that was exactly what I wanted. Perhaps this was one reason I eventually became a psychiatrist.

As a clinician, my professional life became rooted in narrative. Trained to conduct intensive psychotherapy, I made patterns out of the tangled fabric of human lives. I no longer believe in most of these narratives and have even thought of sending out a recall notice to my former patients. However, this would be unnecessary. Most were probably comforted by receiving some sort of explanation for their distress. In any case, they would not remember most of what I told them.

At the other side of narrative lies the future. What could be more exciting than learning the next chapter of a story? Even today, the most interesting patients I see in my hospital clinic are those with the longest histories and the thickest charts. I have cherished the opportunity to see these patients change over time and have experienced many surprises along the way.

About 20 years ago, my hospital held a major conference on BPD. The organizer, my colleague Ron Brown, chose as the theme "The Borderline Patient Over Time." One speaker presented what little was then known on the childhood precursors of the disorder, whereas others described the troubled treatment course of these patients.

I was assigned the task of describing how patients with BPD deal with aging. I looked forward to the literature search, which I expected to enlighten me about an obscure subject. I went to the library and found— *nothing*. Having little of substance to say to the large audience, I was limited to telling a few clinical tales. After the conference, I sat down with Ron and discussed the problem. He suggested we initiate a research project to address these unanswered questions. I did not know it then, but this was the turning point of my career.

I received seed money from the hospital to conduct a formal study. In collaboration with Ron, as well as a research psychologist and an energetic research assistant, our team reevaluated 100 patients with BPD who had been treated 15 years earlier. This research was eventually published, and the main article (Paris et al. 1987) remains my most quoted publication. Even more important for me, this project was the beginning of a serious commitment to research. Having begun my professional life as a clinician-teacher, I had not anticipated that development.

Physicists who work on particle accelerators engage in a struggle for temporal priority that can determine who wins the next Nobel Prize. This is far from the case in psychiatric research. If anything, our situation is precisely the reverse. Given the inherent complexities of mental disorders, we tend to be unsure about the generalizability of our findings. It is positively gratifying when someone else carries out a similar study. As Ron Brown and I were talking, unbeknownst to us, other people were having similar conversations with *their* colleagues. None of them knew what any of the others were planning. This was serendipity indeed!

The first of these landmark studies was carried out by Tom McGlashan at Chestnut Lodge, a hospital outside Washington, D.C. Tom is a clinical scientist well known for work on schizophrenia, and his research benefited from an unusually meticulous and elegant design.

The second study was carried out by Michael Stone at New York State Psychiatric Institute. Mike, a creative clinician and a persistent man, located over 200 former patients with BPD—without any external funds, mostly by using his personal telephone.

At the same time, other studies on the long-term outcome of BPD were being conducted: at Austen Riggs Center in Stockbridge, Massachusetts; at the University of Toronto; and in Oslo, Norway. Remarkably, all obtained strikingly similar results. Because every research project has its own limitations, this powerful consensus added great weight to the conclusions we had reached in Montreal.

After publishing our results, I talked to Tom McGlashan about what further research would be needed to understand the outcome of BPD. He suggested I recontact my original cohort and carry out additional follow-up evaluations every 5 years as the cohort aged. I took his advice and wrote a grant application for a 20-year follow-up process. Discouragingly, the reviewers expressed little confidence in our ability to find the patients in the original study. Why, they asked, would people at that stage of life even want to talk to us? Yet as my colleagues (and my family) will no doubt agree, I am a stubborn man.

Eventually, borrowing from another grant, I found funds to conduct the study. Most of the cohort was indeed locatable. Our ex-patients were happy to hear from us, even keen to tell us how their lives had turned out. The results have now been published (Paris and Zweig-Frank 2001; Zweig-Frank and Paris 2002). This book describes the cohort in much greater detail.

By the 1990s, my research interests in personality disorders grew wider. I conducted a large-scale study of the childhood experiences of patients with personality disorders. I joined a child psychiatry research group studying a population with symptoms that seemed to be precursors of personality disorders. I studied the neurobiological and genetic correlates of personality traits and disorders. I have written about the relationship between culture and personality disorders. The present book aims to bring together all these interests.

Treatment in the Light of Outcome

When I trained in psychiatry and learned to conduct psychotherapy, I was troubled by the slow progress of my patients. The answer I received from my supervisors was always the same: "These things take time." Like Marxists preparing for revolution, or Christians yearning for the second coming, we were taught to wait.

Our teachers claimed it takes at least 5 (or even 10) years of struggle to cure patients with serious personality disorders. They offered no proof for this belief, only anecdotes from their practices. More honestly, one of my teachers openly acknowledged that he was treating patients with BPD for life. In his view, termination would come only when either he or the patient died. No one considered the possibility that in these longer time frames, patients' functioning can improve naturalistically—with or without psychotherapy.

Research on the long-term outcome of personality disorders has documented the importance of naturalistic recovery. If patients get better over time, even without treatment, how can we be sure that long-term therapy is uniquely effective? Virtually all patients in the studies by McGlashan (1986a) and Stone (1990) received long courses of treatment. In contrast, the patients in our Montreal cohort varied enormously in this regard—a few were in long-term therapy, but most received little more than crisis intervention. One cannot validly compare samples from different studies, and true therapeutic benefits could be masked by differing study designs. Yet there was essentially little difference in outcome between any of the BPD cohorts followed for long-term outcome.

Therapy should speed this process of naturalistic recovery. Unfortunately, this does not always happen. Treatment outcome depends on many factors, ranging from diagnosis to past level of functioning. In my own practice, I have had a fair degree of success with a selected group of patients with personality disorders. However, these patients were chosen for treatability, largely on the basis of personal histories showing a capacity for consistent work. Not all patients experience improved functioning—even when the therapist has sufficient skill, talent, and experience.

In the mid-twentieth century, Hans Eysenck (1952) challenged psychotherapists to prove the general efficacy of their methods. Research has since addressed many of the issues he raised. It is now well established that short courses of therapy control acute symptoms more rapidly than does waiting without treatment (see Bergin and Garfield 1994). However, we do not know whether these good results apply to long-term therapy. Eysenck was absolutely right to ask these questions—and he was talking about treatments lasting for only a year or so!

In chronic illness, we aim for care rather than for cure. In acute conditions, such as depression, remotivation and remobilization are often sufficient conditions for recovery (Frank and Frank 1991), but personality disorders require a different approach. Rehabilitative methods used for other chronic diseases provide a good model. We do not aim to "cure" bronchial asthma, peptic ulcer, or rheumatoid arthritis. These patients' conditions can be effectively managed when we ameliorate, rather than eliminate, symptoms and help to achieve a better level of functioning.

Personality disorders are maladaptive exaggerations of normal traits. However, because traits change very slowly, if at all, it should not be surprising that disorders are chronic. Yet this relationship also suggests an approach to management. Therapists can teach patients to understand the adaptive and nonadaptive aspects of their personality and to use these characteristics in positive ways.

In the case of impulsive disorders, therapy can speed recovery by teaching patients to manage problematic traits. Taking the outcome research on BPD into account, Allen Frances (personal communication, 1993) once suggested that patients should be told not to kill themselves because they need to wait only 10 or 15 years to get better. Beyond his irony, Frances was making a serious point: It may be worthwhile to hold on to patients in therapy if we know they will eventually experience improved functioning over time.

Unlike my teachers, I do not claim to know how to cure patients with personality disorders. Instead, I suggest ways to *manage* their treatment. I advocate outpatient therapy and argue against hospitalization—even when patients threaten suicide. A model based on an expectation of chronicity but gradual recovery leads logically to intermittent rather than to continuous interventions. This framework aims to replace grandiose goals with practicality and realism.

The Point of View of This Book

The story of personality disorders begins, as one might expect, in childhood. Although children at risk for personality pathology in adulthood can be identified early on, I do not believe, contrary to received clinical wisdom, that personality disorders are primarily caused by childhood experiences. Instead, I present a model suggesting that children with temperamental problems are more sensitive to life stressors and that interactions between these vulnerabilities and adverse life experiences shape the nature of personality pathology.

Most adult mental disorders do not begin before puberty. However, many have identifiable precursors that are apparent years before diagnosis is possible. These childhood symptoms can be subtle and subclinical, reflecting temperament and traits rather than overt symptoms. Personality disorders are no exception. In view of the instability of childhood symptoms, DSM-IV-TR sets the bar high for making a specific diagnosis before age 18 years. Nonetheless, personality pathology can be reliably identified by middle or late adolescence (Bernstein et al. 1993).

Personality disorders have a waxing and waning course over the years (Grilo et al. 2000). Although they cause much frustration for clinicians in the short run, personality disorders in Cluster B show a gradual improvement over time that could be described as burning out (Paris 2002b). In contrast, personality disorders in Cluster A and Cluster C of Axis II do not seem to improve over time.

In summary, personality pathology has characteristic precursors, a characteristic course, and a characteristic outcome. These relationships between illness and time point to the origins of these disorders and define a framework for conducting effective therapy.

As much as possible, this book is evidence based. In general, I prefer to give more weight to research data than to personal experience. This reflects my belief that good clinical care must be informed by systematic data. However, the study of personality disorders is still in its early stages. At this point, we cannot empirically address many pressing questions. Therefore, I sometimes rely on my experience as a therapist and present clinical vignettes here to illustrate conclusions.

Another limitation to an evidence-based approach derives from problems with the present categories of personality disorder. At best, the DSM-IV-TR classification is provisional—a way of communicating about phenomena that are still poorly understood. Moreover, most research on Axis II has focused on antisocial and borderline personality disorders in Cluster B. This book goes beyond any of these categories, proposing a broader model based on the personality trait dimensions that underlie disorders.

The Purpose of This Book

I have written this book for clinicians who treat patients with personality disorders. The focus is on course: how disorders start in childhood, emerge in adolescence and young adulthood, and sometimes remit in middle age. These patterns underlie my recommendations about therapy. However, this book is not a treatment manual. Readers wanting more details should be referred to other books: I would particularly recommend volumes by John Gunderson (2001) and Marsha Linehan (1993) on the treatment of BPD, as well as a forthcoming book by John Livesley (in press) on the management of all categories of personality disorder.

Although 10 personality disorders are listed in DSM-IV-TR, most research and clinical literature concerns the borderline category, reflecting the fact that patients with BPD are prevalent in practice and present serious challenges in therapy. Much of this book is about BPD, which has been the focus of my own research, but I also present a general theory of personality disorders, along with specific discussion of other categories, showing how each Axis II cluster requires a unique therapeutic approach.

The Structure of This Book

The first three chapters are about the precursors of personality disorders. Chapter 1 ("Time and Illness") offers a broad view of the relationship between time and illness, placing Axis II disorders in a larger context: the childhood precursors and long-term outcome of externalizing, internalizing, and cognitive disorders. Chapter 2 ("Precursors of Personality Disorders") specifically examines the childhood precursors of personality disorders. Chapter 3 ("Borderline Pathology of Childhood") focuses on a particular example, the child with borderline pathology.

The next four chapters are about course and outcome. Chapter 4 ("Personality Disorders in Adulthood") presents a general theory of personality disorders in adult life, pointing to relationships between etiology and chronicity. Chapter 5 ("Long-Term Outcome of Personality Disorders") describes research on the long-term outcome of personality disorders. Chapter 6 ("Patients With Borderline Personality Disorder After 27 Years") provides clinical examples of patients with BPD, drawn from a 27-year follow-up study. Chapter 7 ("Mechanisms of Recovery") discusses the mechanisms of recovery in patients with Cluster B personality disorders.

The last three chapters are about treatment. Chapter 8 ("Course, Prevention, and Management") focuses on the implications of course and outcome for therapy. Chapter 9 ("Suicide and Borderline Personality Disorder") discusses the management of chronic suicidality in BPD. Chapter 10 ("Working With Traits") presents a general model of therapy for personality disorders.

Acknowledgments

I would like to thank several professional colleagues with whom I have enjoyed stimulating research collaborations. The study of children with borderline pathology was carried out by a team that included Jaswant Guzder and Phyllis Zelkowitz. The 15-year follow-up study of patients with BPD was a collaboration with Ron Brown and David Nowlis. The 27-year follow-up study was planned and carried out with Hallie Zweig-Frank.

I would also like thank a series of research assistants who have worked with my team. Marian Van Horne recruited the subjects for the study of children with borderline pathology. Joan Oppenheimer located former patients with BPD for the 15-year follow-up study. Jodi Parnass and Eva Dolenszky relocated them for the 27-year follow-up study. Without their help, I would not have known what happened to the people described in this book.

Finally, I would like to express gratitude to those who agreed to read and provide detailed comments on earlier versions of this manuscript: my wife, Rosalind Paris, and my long-time research colleague, Hallie Zweig-Frank. My librarian, Judy Grossman, demonstrated great skills in finding obscure references.

Some of the ideas in this book have appeared in journal articles. Chapter 3 ("Borderline Pathology of Childhood"), on children with borderline pathology, is a revision of an article in *Psychiatric Clinics of North America* (Paris 2000a). Portions of Chapter 5 ("Long-Term Outcome of Personality Disorders") appeared in *Harvard Review of Psychiatry* (Paris 2002b). Chapter 8 ("Course, Prevention, and Management") is a different version of an article published in *Psychiatric Services* (Paris 2002a).

1

Time and Illness

This chapter is a prelude to the rest of the book. Personality disorders are not essentially different from other types of chronic mental illness. All major forms of psychopathology have characteristic precursors, a characteristic course, and a characteristic outcome.

I examine six aspects of the relationship between time and illness: 1) the nature of chronicity; 2) the continuity of symptoms between childhood and adulthood; 3) the relationship among age at onset, heritability, and chronicity; 4) adolescence and the onset of mental disorders; 5) social sensitivity and the onset of illness; 6) aging and long-term outcome. I draw on data about Axis I and Axis II disorders to illustrate each of these issues.

The Nature of Chronicity

Acute disease is a normal part of living. Everyone falls ill from time to time. Science knows a great deal about the mechanisms of illnesses that come on suddenly. Infectious diseases are the best example. During most of the course of history, many died young because of infections, which were the limiting factor for longevity. Today, a combination of improved public health, vaccines, and antibiotics has given us an extended life span. In developed countries, death is more likely to result from disorders that are chronic and disabling.

Most of the mysteries of modern medicine lie in chronicity. This is because the causes of chronic disease are complex and multifactorial. Genetic vulnerability is usually involved (Nesse and Williams 1994); however, predispositions to chronic illness are associated not with a single gene but with interactions among many genes and are therefore called "complex traits" (McGuffin and Gottesman 1985). These predispositions, by themselves, do not lead to illness but determine thresholds of response to environmental stressors (Falconer 1989). Finally, single stressors rarely cause disease;

1

rather, the cumulative effects of many stressors trigger illness onset (Rutter and Rutter 1993).

Chronic diseases that begin later in life (e.g., arteriosclerosis, essential hypertension, type 2 diabetes mellitus) do not affect reproduction and therefore have not been eliminated by natural selection (Nesse and Williams 1994). Chronic illnesses that begin earlier in life (e.g., bronchial asthma and rheumatoid arthritis) interfere with fertility. Why do the alleles for these illnesses remain prevalent in the population? The most probable explanation is that many genes are involved in vulnerability to disease. Even clearly heritable mental illnesses like schizophrenia, which derive from complex traits, have not disappeared (Meehl 1990).

The course of chronic disease is unique for every patient. Heterogeneity in outcome depends on genetic loadings that modulate severity as well as on degree of exposure to favorable or unfavorable environmental factors (Rutter 1991). However, although every illness is different, physicians still find it useful to organize disease into categories. Classifications of illness become clinically meaningful when they reflect specific etiologies and specific treatments. Although we are long way from understanding the causes of most mental disorders, or of developing therapies specific to each category, describing characteristic patterns of course and outcome is an important first step toward diagnostic validity (Robins and Guze 1970).

Emil Kraepelin was the first psychiatrist to take this approach, one that revolutionized the field. In the nineteenth century, psychiatrists lacked a valid classification of mental illness. Kraepelin (1919) divided psychoses on the basis of outcome: into a deteriorating type (dementia praecox or schizophrenia) and a remitting type (manic depression). Decades later, Robins and Guze (1970) revived these ideas, proposing that *any* valid psychiatric diagnosis should have a characteristic outcome and response to treatment. Their assumption was that illness course should reflect specific biological mechanisms.

Do these principles apply to personality disorders? They definitely do. These conditions emerge early in life, affect functioning over many years, and are quintessentially chronic, but we are just beginning to accumulate data about their etiology. Recent evidence shows that personality disorders have a significant heritable component (Torgersen et al. 2001). However, as is the case for other chronic diseases, these genetic factors are complex (Livesley et al. 1998). There is also strong evidence that psychosocial factors act as precipitants for illness, amplifying personality traits into clinically diagnosable disorders (Paris 1996).

We have a long way to go in developing a valid classification of personality disorders (Livesley, in press). The problem derives from our lack of knowledge about etiology and pathogenesis. Nonetheless, the course and outcome of personality disorders, as well as their response to treatment, give these diagnoses great practical significance. When we describe a patient as antisocial, borderline, schizoid, or avoidant, we make implicit predictions about illness course, as well as about future response to therapy.

Continuity of Symptoms Between Childhood and Adulthood

Mental illness does not usually come "out of the blue," striking down people who have previously been perfectly normal. Of course, this can happen: Adults with happy and untroubled childhoods do develop psychiatric disorders (Rutter 1989). However, a careful study of the precursors of mental disorders often identifies traits during childhood that *precede* overt symptoms in adulthood. We may only need to look carefully enough.

The precursors of mental disorders usually consist of subclinical symptoms or behavioral characteristics. Traits that deviate markedly from normality are likely to be rooted in genetic variations and temperament (Kagan 1989). By and large, when a disorder eventually develops, the traits underlying pathology will have been stable over time (Kagan 1994).

These principles have been supported by research findings. A large-scale and long-term follow-up study of patients from a British child psychiatry clinic (Zeitlin 1986) found that only a minority eventually developed mental disorders in adulthood. The most likely explanation is that many children attending psychiatric clinics have less severe symptoms, such as minor degrees of oppositional behavior and learning difficulties, that are not consistent predictors of adult illness.

In contrast, severely disturbed children are at significant risk for psychopathology later in life. In a book edited by Hechtman (1996), entitled *Do They Grow Out of It?*, a number of experts reviewed the course of conduct disorder, attention-deficit/hyperactivity disorder (ADHD), mood disorders, and anxiety disorders from childhood into adulthood. The answer to the question posed in the title was: *usually not.*

Confusion about the childhood precursors of adult illness results from the imprecise way we classify disorders. Diagnostic categories, both in children and in adults, tend to overlap, producing "comorbid" patterns. We can avoid this problem by examining *traits* that account for commonalities between different categories of illness.

One of the most basic of all trait dimensions involves the dichotomy between disturbances in behavior versus inner distress. In children, clinicians make the distinction between *externalizing* and *internalizing* symptoms (Achenbach and McConaughy 1997). Some children react to stressors through impulsive actions, whereas others react through internal suffering. A similar distinction can be applied to adults. In a striking study, Krueger (1999) applied factor analysis to all the mental disorders in DSM and showed that most comorbidity patterns across categories can be accounted for by only two dimensions: one externalizing, the other internalizing. (This distinction does not account for the cognitive dimension of psychopathology, seen in disorders such as schizophrenia.)

No dichotomy is absolute. Externalizing and internalizing symptoms can and do coexist (Zahn-Waxler et al. 2000), but when one type is predominant, we tend to observe consistency over time. Externalizing disorders in childhood tend to be precursors of impulsive disorders in adulthood, whereas internalizing disorders in childhood tend to be precursors of mood and anxiety disorders in adulthood. Abnormal behavioral patterns in childhood can also be precursors of cognitive disorders in adulthood.

I will illustrate the childhood precursors of adult pathology using this division into externalizing, internalizing, and cognitive disorders.

Externalizing Disorders

Conduct disorder is a direct precursor of an Axis II disorder. The pioneering work of Robins (1966) showed that about one-third of children with conduct disorder will meet criteria for antisocial personality by age 18. In many ways, the personality disorder is simply a continuation of the childhood symptoms. At the same time, conduct symptoms can also be precursors of other mental disorders. Although two-thirds do not develop antisocial personality, these children are also at risk for substance abuse and mood disorders as adults (Zoccolillo et al. 1992). As we will see, they are also at risk for other categories of personality disorder.

When conduct disorder is severe and of early onset, it is particularly likely to lead to sequelae (Moffit 1993). Extreme temperaments lead to maladaptive behavioral patterns that tend to continue, even in more favorable environments (Kagan 1994). Moreover, because these behavioral symptoms are difficult for parents, teachers, and peers to manage, children with conduct disorders are more likely to be rejected and/or mistreated, which leads to negative feedback loops (Rutter and Smith 1995). In contrast, behavioral symptoms that are less rooted in temperament are more likely to remit when a child is exposed to a different environment (Rutter 1989).

Conduct disorder can lead to different outcomes because, like so many other categories in psychiatry, it describes a heterogeneous group of patients. Some are responding primarily to unfavorable family environments

(Robins 1966), whereas others have symptoms that are strongly rooted in temperamental vulnerabilities (Cadoret et al. 1995). Moffit (1993) described these two pathways as "life-course persistent" and "adolescence-limited" antisocial behavior.

Some delinquent adolescents have family histories of impulsive disorders and have been irritable and difficult to manage from their earliest years. These adolescents are the ones most likely to go on to develop adult antisocial personality and/or substance abuse. In contrast, adolescents who do not have such family histories, and who develop conduct disorder for the first time after puberty, have a better prognosis. In adolescence-limited antisocial behavior, inconsistent parenting and deviant peer relations maintain symptoms (Patterson and Yoerger 1997). Adolescents with these problems must have *some* degree of trait impulsivity to react in the ways they do (Moeller et al. 2001) but probably lack the temperamental abnormalities seen in those with the life-course persistent type. Thus, most delinquent adolescents with a late onset of problematic behavior "straighten out" by young adulthood (Rutter and Smith 1995).

These patterns suggest a general model for personality disorders. Adults who develop Axis II disorders may have had abnormal temperamental characteristics from an early age. Those who lack such temperamental vulnerabilities would be less likely to have this trajectory.

Mental disorders are not only a product of temperament. Although behavioral genetic studies (Plomin et al. 2000) show that almost all mental illnesses have a heritable component, the same research shows the importance of environmental variance in psychopathology. Twin studies measure whether environmental effects are "shared" (i.e., related to growing up in a particular family) or "unshared" (i.e., not related to growing up in a particular family).

Unshared environmental effects are seen in almost every mental illness (Paris 1999). Conduct disorder is a notable exception to the rule, with a large contribution from the shared environment (Cadoret et al. 1995). This supports the principle that dysfunctional families are important for the development of conduct symptoms (Lykken 1995; Robins 1966).

On the other hand, dysfunctional families produce different symptoms in different children. Those who are temperamentally extroverted and impulsive are more likely to develop conduct symptoms (Moeller et al. 2001). Children with a highly introverted temperament are protected against developing conduct disorder, even under the most adverse conditions (Kagan 1994). As we will see, temperamental differences may explain why a wide range of personality disorders are associated with similar adversities.

The temperamental variability behind antisocial behavior can be identified surprisingly early in life. In a landmark longitudinal study (Caspi et al.

1996), a cohort of children underwent, at age 3, a standard assessment that lasted only 90 minutes. When children who had been noted to have unusually high levels of impulsive and irritable behavior were assessed again at age 18, they were found to be at greater risk for antisocial personality. In the same study, children with unusually withdrawn behavior at age 3 were found to be at greater risk for depression at 18. These striking findings have recently been replicated (Stevenson and Goodman 2001).

These findings should not be interpreted as meaning that every impulsive child will develop a personality disorder. As Lykken (1995) has emphasized, these children require more parental control; if reared carefully by their families, they need not end up in a psychiatric clinic.

The prevalence of conduct disorder also varies with social setting and with culture (Rutter and Smith 1995). Youths with adolescence-limited conduct disorder often become delinquent when they join deviant peer groups, but remission can occur when the environment changes (Moffitt 1993). This helps to explain why social programs can be successful and why naturalistic recovery from late-onset conduct disorder is common once adolescents leave their families and take on adult social roles.

ADHD, the other main externalizing disorder of childhood, is also a precursor of adult illness. The symptoms of the childhood disorder can continue into adult life (Barkley 1998). ADHD also carries an increased long-term risk for antisocial personality and substance abuse (Weiss and Hechtman 1993). The relationship between childhood ADHD and other personality disorders is weaker, and Soloff and Millward (1983) failed to find any link with adult borderline personality disorder. Moreover, children with ADHD are most likely to present clinically when they also have conduct symptoms (Rutter 1989). It is therefore not clear whether ADHD itself or comorbid conduct disorder is the precursor for adult externalizing disorders.

Recently, as ADHD has garnered a great deal of attention among clinicians and in the media, there has been some tendency to explain too much by this diagnosis. In clinical practice, I have seen typical cases of personality disorder in which impulsive behaviors are attributed to adult ADHD. However, it is often difficult to determine whether adults were truly hyperactive as children; one needs hard evidence, particularly from school records, to make a firm diagnosis (Weiss and Hechtman 1993). We need community studies to determine how many adults with ADHD also have personality disorders.

One of the most striking findings of research regarding the roots of externalizing disorders is that predispositions to alcoholism and drug abuse can be observed in childhood. The sons of early onset alcoholics are at high risk for developing the same disorder (Goodwin and Warnock 1991).

Those who may later develop alcoholism may have characteristic personality trait profiles, with high levels of stimulus seeking (Kish 1971). Conrod et al. (2000) have shown that adolescents who become excited when they drink (as measured by increased heart rate) are more likely to develop alcoholism as adults. These physiological markers can be measured before serious clinical problems emerge. Moreover, those who actually begin heavy drinking early in adolescence tend to continue, whereas those who begin drinking later in life, often in response to stressful circumstances, find it easier to stop (Goodwin and Warnock 1991; Schuckit and Smith 1996).

Substance abuse, particularly when it begins in adolescence, shares impulsive traits with other externalizing disorders, such as conduct disorder (Goodwin and Warnock 1991). An early onset of drug and alcohol abuse tends to be comorbid with Cluster B personality disorders (Bernstein et al. 1993). The predisposition to abuse substances may be one of several factors in the background of patients who develop impulsive personality disorders. And when substance abuse does develop, it makes the course of those disorders more severe (Links et al. 1995).

Internalizing Disorders

Although mood and anxiety disorders are highly prevalent in adults, their childhood precursors are not always apparent. Internalizing symptoms in childhood may not present clinically, given that they do not cause behavioral disruption and do not alarm parents and teachers. If moody and nervous children who are quiet and do well in school are not referred, these disorders will go unrecognized in a large number of people (Wu et al. 2001).

Whereas most children seen in child clinics are boys, adult psychiatric patients include a disproportionate number of women. Internalizing symptoms are more common in girls (Achenbach and McConaughy 1997), and adult disorders associated with internalizing symptoms are also more frequent in women (Weissman and Klerman 1985). However, at later stages of development, help-seeking is determined by inner suffering rather than by behavioral disruption (Weissman et al. 1997).

Depressive or anxious symptoms during childhood can be precursors of affective and/or anxiety disorders later in life. Although it was once thought that depression in childhood was rare or nonexistent, this disorder may begin in childhood (Harrington et al. 1996); when it does, it is more likely to recur later in life (Zahn-Waxler et al. 2000). Follow-up studies of adolescent depression (Fombonne et al. 2001; Weissman et al. 1999) have documented unusually high rates of recurrence over time, as well as increases in the ultimate risk for completed suicide.

Mood disorders can present with only one episode in a lifetime or be chronic with frequent relapses. Depressions that are severe, that begin early in life, and that recur over time have a stronger heritable component (McGuffin et al. 1996; Sullivan et al. 2000). In contrast, depressions that are mild, begin later in life, and do not recur may be responses to unfavorable life circumstances (Kendler and Gardner 1998).

Unlike depression, manic-like phenomena in childhood are associated with externalizing symptoms, but the question of whether true mania begins before adolescence remains highly controversial (Weckerly 2002). Because it is difficult to distinguish manic irritability and distractibility from conduct disorder or ADHD (Beiderman et al. 1996a), we need to follow such patients into adulthood to be sure about the diagnosis.

Mood and anxiety disorders overlap, so much so that they may even be considered as a single group (Goldberg 2000). Depression and anxiety could therefore have common precursors and reflect a common temperamental vulnerability. In general, internalizing disorders are related to traits of *neuroticism*, a concept that describes increased levels of emotional reactivity (McCrae and Costa 1999).

Mood and anxiety disorders that are chronic are more likely to show increased comorbidity with personality disorders in adulthood. It has been consistently shown that early onset dysthymia is associated with Cluster B disorders (Pepper et al. 1995; Riso et al. 1996) and that patients with anxiety disorders often meet criteria for Cluster C personality disorders (Mavissakalian et al. 1993). For this reason, a childhood onset of mood and anxiety symptoms may constitute a precursor of Axis II disorders.

Cognitive Disorders

One would expect a disease such as schizophrenia, with its strong genetic component, to be associated with unusual traits or symptoms during childhood. Yet in spite of much research, the precise nature of the relationship remains elusive. Schizophrenia with a later onset is less likely to have shown symptoms in childhood (Palmer et al. 2001). Again, an early onset of disease is associated with chronicity.

A wide range of abnormalities can precede schizophrenia (Sobin et al. 2001), even including conduct disorder (Ricks and Berry 1970). Studies of high-risk populations such as children who have schizophrenic parents (Erlenmeyer-Kimling et al. 2000) elicit subtle but perceptible precursors, involving "soft" neurological signs and/or neuropsychological abnormalities, such as clumsiness, movement disorders, and gait disturbances. Some of these signs can be detected by observing home movies of children who later develop schizophrenia (Walker et al. 1994).

Research on the precursors of schizophrenia also sheds light on the origins of the Cluster A personality disorders lying in the schizophrenic spectrum. Although many patients with schizophrenia do not have affected first-degree relatives (Murray and Van Os 1998), genetic and biological markers are more consistently observed when patients with Cluster A disorders are included in studies (Kendler et al. 1981; Kendler 1995). Some of these children at risk never cross the boundary into psychosis, developing into adults with schizoid or schizotypal personality disorders (Erlenmeyer-Kimling et al. 2000).

Age of Onset, Heritability, and Chronicity

At this point, I would like to introduce two important principles. First, the earlier an illness starts, the more likely it is to become severe and chronic, whereas the later in life an illness begins, the more likely it is to remit. Second, early onset chronic diseases also have a larger genetic component than those whose onset comes later in life. These relationships between age of onset, heritability, and chronicity have been documented for a wide range of medical illnesses (Childs 2000), including common diseases such as duodenal ulcer, non–insulin-dependent diabetes mellitus, Crohn's disease, and gout.

These principles can also be shown to apply to psychiatric illness (see review in Paris 1999). Many disorders beginning early in life, such as autism, childhood psychoses, and the more severe forms of conduct disorder and ADHD, have a large genetic component. Diseases that often begin in adolescence, such as schizophrenia and bipolar illness, also have a moderate to large genetic component. Diseases beginning later in life, such as single episodes of unipolar depression, tend to have a weaker genetic load and a stronger environmental contribution.

Course of illness further illuminates this triangular relationship among age of onset, heritability, and chronicity. Although rapid recovery from acute episodes of illness points to environmental determinants, failure to recover points to genetic vulnerability. Thus, the course of a disorder provides clues about causes.

To understand the causes of most mental disorders, we can apply a stress-diathesis model (Monroe and Simons 1991), in which biological predispositions determine susceptibility to illness, whereas environmental stressors determine symptom onset. When biological predispositions are predominant, environmental stressors may serve only to tip over a delicate balance.

When biological predispositions are weak, illness will occur only in the presence of strong environmental stressors.

Lykken (1995) applied this type of model to the etiology of antisocial personality disorder. Three genotypes lead to different types of interactions. Children with easy-to-socialize temperaments can do well even with relatively incompetent parents. In contrast, hard-to-socialize children may become antisocial unless their parents are highly competent and/or the children are provided with other sources of socialization. Average children will not become antisocial unless their parents are incompetent *and* they lack other socializing influences.

Thus, genotypes and temperament help explain why different children develop different symptoms when exposed to similar adversities. Moreover, predispositions, not environmental stressors, determine the specific nature of the symptoms that emerge—whether externalizing, internalizing, or cognitive disorders (Kagan 1994). Similarly, temperament can account for the fact that different types of personality disorders evolve in patients who are exposed to similar adversities.

Adolescence and the Onset of Disorder

Even when mental disorders have childhood precursors, overt clinical symptoms often present for the first time in adolescence or early adulthood. This age at onset is typical for schizophrenia, bipolar disorder, and substance abuse and is also common in mood and anxiety disorders. Personality disorders can also be clinically diagnosed beginning in the adolescent or young adult years. Why should illness begin at this stage of development—not earlier, or later?

One possibility that has been suggested is that adverse early experiences can produce delayed effects that emerge later in development. This concept, initiated by Freud, characterizes the developmental theory of Erikson (1950). In this model, success or failure at each stage of life depends on how well previous stages have been mastered. Similarly, attachment theory (Bowlby 1969) hypothesizes that adult symptoms develop from early insecurity in relationships with caretakers.

However, contemporary research casts doubt on any simple correspondence between childhood experience and adult psychopathology. I have reviewed this complex subject in detail in an earlier book (Paris 2000c), reaching conclusions similar to those held by senior researchers in child development (e.g., Rutter and Rutter 1993). The interested reader may wish to refer to these books, but two general conclusions emerge from the literature. First, although research has consistently demonstrated that adversities early in development are associated with psychopathology, a vast body of evidence suggests that these events have greater effects on those who are temperamentally vulnerable (Rutter 1989). Second, although repeated and continuous adverse experiences are most likely to cause symptoms, most children demonstrate a surprising level of resilience to stressors such as trauma, neglect, family dysfunction, and social disadvantage (Rutter 1987a).

Let us consider another alternative: Can the onset of mental disorders in adolescence be explained by biological changes? If genes are present from the moment of conception, whereas diseases start years later, we have to hypothesize *sleeper effects*, in which genes are turned on or expressed only at a later point in development (Weinberger 1987). The most dramatic example of these effects is dementia, which can lie in wait for a lifetime before striking a vulnerable individual. Although Alzheimer's disease has a heritable component (Small et al. 1995), its symptoms become apparent only after age 50 or later. Nonetheless, researchers have identified subtle cognitive deficits that can be identified prior to the onset of disease (Skoog 2000).

The brain undergoes major rewiring during adolescence. One current theory about schizophrenia hypothesizes an association with early brain injury (McNeil et al. 2000), with effects becoming apparent only years later. Genetic vulnerability to schizophrenia might cause an abnormal response to injury affecting the migration of neurons (Weinberger 1987), but the resulting neural misconnections could be masked by extensive neuronal growth in early childhood, connections that are "pruned" in adolescence. This *synaptic pruning* could uncover abnormalities occurring earlier in development (Keshavan et al. 1994).

Another possible mechanism involves hormonal changes that occur in adolescence. Increases in oxytocin levels after puberty have a relationship to increased rates of depression in pubescent girls (Frank and Young 2000). However, the relationship between hormonal levels and psychological distress in adolescence is complex (Kaufman et al. 2001) and the direction of causality unclear.

Finally, let us examine the concept of "adolescent turmoil." My generation of clinicians was taught that for a combination of biological, psychological, and social reasons, adolescence is *usually* a time of turmoil. However, a classical study of asymptomatic high school students (Offer and Offer 1975) showed that the vast majority pass through this stage of development without undergoing major disturbances. Although adolescents may undergo minor degrees of upset, this period is more stressful for some and less stressful for others. Most likely, a susceptible minority, with vulnerabilities that interfere with developmental tasks, have more difficulty with the transition.

Social Sensitivity and Onset of Illness

Mental disorders do not develop in a cultural vacuum. Their onset, course, and outcome are influenced by social context.

Some disorders are *socially sensitive*, whereas others are relatively *insensitive*. I define this term by the presence or absence of effects from the sociocultural context on the prevalence and course of illness. The most prominent socially sensitive disorders are substance abuse (Helzer and Canino 1992), eating disorders (Szmukler et al. 1995), antisocial personality (Lykken 1995), and borderline personality (Paris 1996), all of which are characterized by externalizing symptoms, and all of which have been shown to vary widely in prevalence with time and circumstance. Some internalizing disorders, such as unipolar depression, also demonstrate a fair degree of social sensitivity, as shown by recent increases in the prevalence of depression among the young (Weissman et al. 1996). In contrast, schizophrenia, with its stronger biological component and a relatively constant cross-cultural prevalence around the world (Gottesman 1991), seems to be relatively *socially insensitive*, although its course and outcome vary greatly with social context (Murphy 1982).

Socially sensitive disorders tend to show an increased prevalence under conditions of sociocultural change. Epidemiological research in North America and Europe (Rutter and Smith 1995) has demonstrated striking increases in prevalence over recent decades in many categories (substance abuse, depression, and impulsive personality disorders) that affect young people. These "cohort effects" describe increases in prevalence for disorders in specific age groups. Only social change can explain effects occurring over relatively short periods of time (Millon 1993; Paris 1996).

Cross-cultural studies support the concept of social sensitivity. For example, societies such as Taiwan (Hwu et al. 1989) and Japan (Sato and Takeichi 1993) have a lower prevalence of substance abuse and antisocial personality among the young than most Western societies. Although such differences might be partly genetic, they are not seen in all East Asian societies: South Korea has a high prevalence of both substance abuse and antisocial behavior (Lee et al. 1987).

The distinction between *traditional* and *modern* societies is essential for understanding the role of sociocultural factors in mental disorders. This terminology has been used by social scientists (Inkeles and Smith 1974; Lerner 1958) to describe two general types of social structure. Traditional societies have slow rates of social change and have intergenerational continuity, whereas modern societies have rapid social change and have intergenerational discontinuity.

During most of human history, people lived in extended families, villages, and tribes. They rarely traveled very far from home, even in the course of a lifetime. The few who did not fit in might leave and search for a niche elsewhere. Most stayed put, doing the same work as their parents and their grandparents, learning the necessary skills from relatives who raised them. Nor did people have to search very far to find intimate relationships. Marriage was arranged early, with partners chosen from the same or from neighboring communities.

Consider, in contrast, the tasks required of adolescents in a modern society. They are expected to spend years learning how to function as adults, to take on different roles, and to "find themselves," developing a unique identity. Young people rarely do the same work as their parents and have to learn necessary skills from strangers. Families may not even understand the nature of their children's careers. Finally, young people are expected to find their own mates. Because there is no guarantee that this search will be successful, the young need to deal with the vicissitudes of mistaken choices, hurtful rejections, and intermittent loneliness.

Adolescence has different meanings in traditional versus modern societies. Although puberty is universal, adolescence, as a separate developmental stage, can be seen as a social construction. Throughout most of history, young people assumed adult roles early in life. Adolescence as a stage emerges in societies that expect the younger generation to postpone maturity to learn complex skills and to develop an identity different from that of their parents.

Not everyone is cut out for this challenge. Adolescence is stressful for those who are vulnerable to stress. In traditional societies, young people are protected by being provided social roles and supportive networks. In modern societies, adolescents must manage with lower levels of protection and support.

As moderns, we value individualism and would be thoroughly miserable in a traditional society. Most of us manage the transition to adulthood with success, but modernity is a problem for those who are temperamentally vulnerable. How can impulsive adolescents choose a career when models and guidance are unavailable? How can moody adolescents deal with the cruelty and rejection of peers in the absence of a predictable environment? How can shy adolescents find intimate relationships when they can barely introduce themselves to a stranger?

Youth is not a happy time for everyone. Western culture is built on energy, innovation, and an appetite for change. Young people have to establish themselves in the world, and their choices have become increasingly complex. Therefore, it should not be surprising that the prevalence of mental disorders rises in late adolescence, peaks in young adulthood, and then falls off in middle age. Community surveys (Robins and Regier 1991; Tohen et al. 2000) consistently show that cohorts between ages 20 and 40 have the highest rate of psychological symptoms.

In this context, it also should not be surprising that adolescence and young adulthood are the ages when personality disorders are usually first diagnosed (Westen and Chang 2000). These conditions may have childhood precursors related to temperamental vulnerability, but overt symptoms emerge with exposure to stressors associated with coming of age.

Aging and Long-Term Outcome

There is a common prejudice that youth is a happy time and that later life is inevitably disillusioning. The "midlife crisis," a response to a narrowing of life's possibilities around age 40, is a social construction that reflects modern attitudes toward aging. Research shows that for most people, growing older is a positive experience. In a long-term follow-up study of a community cohort, Vaillant and Mukamal (2001) found that successful aging was common, although a good outcome clearly depended on prior psychological health.

In contrast, patients with serious mental disorders may not age well. Some are never able to find meaningful work. Many suffer from the outcomes of family breakdown. Some remain lonely all their lives. These phenomena are particularly common in patients with personality disorders (Skodol et al. 2002).

Community surveys (Robins and Regier 1991) show an overall reduction in psychiatric symptoms in late adulthood. In part, this lower prevalence is due to the remission of symptoms. Many mental disorders begin in late adolescence or youth, produce serious effects for a number of years, and then gradually remit. This constitutes their *natural course*. As I will show, striking improvements over time have been observed for patients with substance abuse, eating disorders, impulsive spectrum personality disorders, and even schizophrenia. However, patients with other disorders do not improve, and a few even get worse with age.

To illustrate the long-term outcome of mental disorders, I will once again organize the discussion around internalizing, externalizing, and cognitive disorders, considering which symptoms are most (or least) likely to improve, and the possible mechanisms influencing remission.

Externalizing Disorders

Improvement over time is striking in disorders characterized by impulsivity. This process is well documented in substance abuse. The highest prevalence occurs among the young (Robins and Regier 1991), and symptoms tend to remit in middle age. Although alcoholism is famous for chronicity, many of those with alcoholism eventually control abuse, showing a dramatic social recovery even when they have been drinking heavily for a long time (Vaillant 1995). Among those who fail to control their alcoholism, longevity is decreased (Liskow et al. 2000). Similar patterns of recovery are seen in other forms of substance abuse, but when opiates are the drug of choice, early death is common (Vaillant 1992; Hser et al. 2001).

Eating disorders also tend to improve with time. Bulimia nervosa, an impulsive spectrum disorder, rarely continues into middle age. In a long-term follow-up study (Keel et al. 1999), only 10% of patients still met criteria for the disorder, although 30% continued to have subclinical problems with eating behavior. The pattern in anorexia nervosa, a condition associated with compulsive (internalizing) rather than impulsive traits, is different, and 10% of patients with severe illness die prematurely (Crow et al. 1999).

Criminality is another impulsive pattern that tends to level out by age 40 (Arbodela-Flores and Holley 1991; Yochelson and Samenow 1976). Antisocial behaviors are also associated with a higher rate of unnatural deaths, as documented in a 50-year follow-up study of delinquent boys (Laub and Vaillant 2000) and in a follow-up study of adults with antisocial personality disorder (Black et al. 1997).

Thus, in various clinical pictures associated with externalizing symptoms, we see improvement over time. Chapter 5 describes similar levels of remission in Cluster B personality disorders.

Internalizing Disorders

Kraepelin (1919) observed that mood disorders are remitting rather than deteriorating. He separated them from schizophrenia on the basis of better functioning between episodes, as well as their better prognosis. Yet some depressed patients never recover fully (Kessing et al. 1998), and follow-up studies have observed troublingly high rates of relapse (Shea et al. 1992). Although bipolar illness is not an internalizing disorder, its outcome is even more problematic: In spite of an intermittent course, patients do not recover as they age, and their illness may become progressively resistant to treatment (Shulman et al. 1992). Winokur and Tsuang (1996) conducted a 40-year follow-up study of 100 patients with bipolar illness and 225 patients with unipolar illness who had been admitted to a state hospital, and they found that most continued to have serious symptoms. Mania was associated with a particularly high morbidity: The suicide rate was 9.3%, and total unnatural deaths reached 18.5%. The rates for unipolar depression were not much better: For suicide the rate was 8%, and for unnatural deaths, 15.4%. Although a community sample of depressed patients would have yielded more optimistic results than were obtained from this hospitalized sample, mortality figures in patients with depression (Wulsin et al. 1999) demonstrate a decrease in overall longevity, largely because of a correlation with cardiovascular illness.

Anxiety disorders are also more chronic than psychiatrists had originally thought. In a follow-up study of 145 patients with panic disorder or generalized anxiety disorder (Seivewright et al. 1998), 60% recovered after 5 years, but 40% did not. As Chapter 5 shows, patients with Axis II disorders in Cluster C, which are frequently associated with internalizing symptoms, also continue to show serious defects in functioning well into middle age.

Cognitive Disorders

The long-term outcome of schizophrenia is well-documented. Kraepelin (1919) originally coined the term *dementia praecox* to describe a form of psychosis that begins early in life and then leads to social deterioration over subsequent decades. This course is most likely in patients in whom illness begins early; a later onset of illness is associated with a milder course and less chronicity (Palmer et al. 2001).

Nonetheless, follow-up research in Europe and the United States shows that many patients with schizophrenia get better with time. When these observations were published, they came as a surprise. Our perceptions were distorted by seeing the sickest patients, who remain in the treatment system, whereas recovered patients disappear from view.

A recent international collaborative study (Harrison et al. 2001) reported that about 50% of patients with schizophrenia are found to have had favorable outcomes when assessed 15–25 years later. Studies in Switzerland (Bleuler 1974; Ciompi 1980), Germany (Huber et al. 1975), and Japan (Ogawa et al. 1987) that followed patients with schizophrenia for decades all found more than half of the patients to be improved or fully recovered. Harding et al. (1987), in a follow-up study of schizophrenic patients in Vermont and Maine, found that about half of the cohort recovered over time, with many no longer meeting criteria for schizophrenia. The subjects fell into three more or less equal groups (Harding and Keller 1998): "loners" (who did not maintain social recovery); "self-regulators" (who successfully adapted); and "niche people" (who survived in sheltered environments). Finally, Winokur and Tsuang (1996) reported similar findings in a state hospital sample of 200 patients with schizophrenia followed for 40 years: 20% were asymptomatic at follow-up evaluation, whereas 35% maintained "reasonable" functioning. However, not all patients lived to the age at which improvement might be expected. The suicide rate was 9%, with all unnatural deaths combined reaching 16.7%. (In Chapter 5, we find similar figures for personality disorders.)

Improvement in schizophrenia usually occurs after the age of 50. Moreover, remission is far from complete and affects positive more than negative symptoms (Gottesman 1991). Yet when those with schizophrenia have fewer delusions or hallucinations as they age, they are better able to survive in the community, albeit on a marginal level.

A dramatic example of this type of outcome was described in a biography (Nasar 1998) of John Foster Nash, the Nobel Prize–winning mathematician. (This excellent book was later turned into a successful film, which unfortunately had only a vague resemblance to the facts of Nash's life.) Although he was strange and eccentric, Nash made major contributions to economic game theory in his twenties. After developing paranoid schizophrenia at age 30, Nash spent many years in a delusional state, receiving "messages" from extraterrestrials about creating a world government. Nash was unable to work, even when the disease began to remit in his fifties. By age 66, however, he had recovered sufficiently to accept his Nobel Prize and even to lecture about his ideas. As he approached 70, Nash continued to experience occasional hallucinations and delusional thoughts but had trained himself to ignore them.

The long-term outcome of schizophrenia depends both on genetic loading and environmental factors. This principle is demonstrated by a well-known case. The "Genain quadruplets" are a group of genetically identical women who were born to a schizophrenic mother in 1930. When originally studied (Rosenthal 1968), all four were diagnosed as schizophrenic by the criteria used at the time, although one, "Myra," had a clinical picture closer to schizotypal personality disorder. In a follow-up study at age 66 (Mirsky et al. 2000), all the quadruplets showed some degree of improvement over time, but Myra had an unusually good outcome. Whereas none of the others were ever able to function in normal social roles, Myra worked as a secretary for much of her life, was married, and had two sons. We do not know why Myra did better than her sisters, but given that her genetic profile was identical, she may have had a different developmental history.

Cross-cultural research demonstrates that environmental factors affect the outcome of schizophrenia. The disease has a very different course in developing countries than in the Western world (Murphy 1982). In traditional societies, the disorder tends to be more episodic, with less loss of social functioning. These settings do not make the same demands as people experience in an industrial or postindustrial world. In an agrarian society, one can more easily find a nondemanding social role and can be supported by extended family and community without having to deal with high-intensity interactions with other people. Many patients with schizophrenia (and schizotypal personality disorder) whom I have known would make good shepherds, but they do not find this kind of work in a modern city.

The bad news is that many patients with schizophrenia continue to have negative symptoms, even when their positive symptoms remit (Harding and Keller 1998). Thus, the long-term outcome of this illness leaves a residue that very much resembles schizotypal personality disorder. As we see in Chapter 5, that group of patients does not recover with time.

We do not know why schizophrenia eventually remits. One possibility is that neurotransmitter functions become more stable over time. Another is that patients, especially those with milder illness, may eventually find social roles. As we see later in this book, both mechanisms play a role in the outcome of personality disorders.

2

Precursors of Personality Disorders

Personality disorders have all the characteristics that point to childhood precursors. They begin early in life, are chronic, and have severe effects on functioning. However, childhood precursors of adult illness need not consist of diagnosable disorders. Rather, they usually consist of trait profiles that are not by themselves pathological.

Personality Traits and Axis II Clusters

Personality disorders, as defined in DSM-IV-TR (American Psychiatric Association 2000), begin early in life. However, symptoms in children are not the same as those in adults. As discussed in Chapter 1, these commonalities reflect broad dimensions associated with externalizing, internalizing, and cognitive symptoms. Thus, the vulnerabilities that precede overt disorders will be apparent as *traits*.

Personality traits describe individual differences in behavior, emotion, and cognition, resulting from interactions between temperament and life experience (Rutter 1987b). These characteristics can be identified early in childhood (Rothbart et al. 2000). Although trait profiles need not be pathological, they can be associated with an increased risk for disorders.

Chapter 4 examines the classification of personality traits in more detail. At this point, it is sufficient to note that each category of Axis II disorder is associated with a characteristic dimensional profile (Costa and Widiger 2001). When categories overlap (as they often do), the commonalities tend to reflect common traits (Nurnberg et al. 1994). Most Axis II comorbidity falls within the three Axis II clusters (Oldham et al. 1992), suggesting that these clusters reflect broad trait dimensions. In fact, the three Axis II clusters correspond rather closely to the broad dimensions of psychopathology described in Chapter 1: *externalizing* (Cluster B), *internalizing* (Cluster C), and *cognitive* (Cluster A).

Therefore, I organize the discussion of childhood precursors around these Axis II clusters. I prefer to use older terminology introduced in DSM-III (American Psychiatric Association 1980): *odd*, *dramatic*, and *anxious*, to refer to the three clusters. (This language is more descriptive, unlike the non-committal terminology of DSM-IV [American Psychiatric Association 1994], which labeled the clusters only as A, B, and C.) The A (*odd*) cluster is characterized by high levels of introversion and/or unusual cognitions. The B (*dramatic*, or, as I prefer, *impulsive*) cluster is associated with impulsivity as well as affective instability. The C (*anxious*) cluster is characterized by social anxiety or an unusual need for control. These are the trait profiles most likely to be identifiable in childhood prior to the onset of personality disorders.

Childhood Precursors of Odd Cluster Disorders

The three categories of personality disorder in Cluster A—schizoid, schizotypal, and paranoid—fall in the "schizophrenic spectrum," that is, they derive from predispositions similar to schizophrenia but do not lead to overt psychotic symptoms. Several lines of evidence confirm these links. Behavior genetic studies show that, as a group, Cluster A personality disorders share a common heritable component (Torgersen et al. 2000). In family studies, when all spectrum disorders are combined, heritability coefficients are almost always greater than they are for schizophrenia alone (Kendler et al. 1993).

Schizotypal personality and schizophrenia have a particularly close connection. These two disorders share many negative (and a few positive) symptoms, as well as biological markers and family histories of disorder (Siever and Davis 1991). In the past, schizotypal personality disorder was categorized as a form of schizophrenia: In Bleuler's (1950) terminology, patients with negative symptoms and no positive symptoms were described as having the "simple" type. Schizoid and paranoid personality disorders do not have as close a relationship with psychosis, but both run in the same families in which schizophrenia does (Kendler et al. 1993). When these disorders are studied separately, it is apparent that both have a moderate heritable component (Torgersen et al. 2000).

The boundaries between the three disorders in Cluster A are somewhat unclear, and there is some overlap (Nurnberg et al. 1994). The childhood precursors of these conditions could also be similar. In a follow-up study of

32 children with schizoid traits (Wolff et al. 1991), 24 developed schizo-typal disorder in adulthood and 2 went on to develop schizophrenia.

We do not know why some patients develop full-blown psychosis while others develop personality disorders. Meehl (1990) has suggested that schizotypal traits are more widely distributed in the population than psychosis. Patients with psychosis might carry a higher genetic load, whereas a lower load could be associated with the partial impairment seen in personality disorders.

On the other hand, identical genes do not produce identical results. As shown by the story of the Genain quadruplets described in Chapter 1, environmental factors may determine whether individuals develop schizophrenia or a Cluster A personality disorder. We do not know precisely what these factors are. One possible mechanism could involve fetal or perinatal brain injury (Weinberger 1987). Some patients with schizotypal traits stay on the "right" side of the psychotic border by avoiding environments to which they are particularly sensitive (McGlashan 1991). These patients have difficulty with circumstances that require emotional expressiveness and may do better in settings that are structured and predictable.

Childhood Precursors of Impulsive Cluster Disorders

Antisocial Personality Disorder

We know more about the precursors of antisocial personality disorder (ASPD) than any other category on Axis II. The data were collected by Lee Robins, a sociologist at Washington University in St. Louis, in the 1950s. She took excellent advantage of a rare opportunity to reevaluate a large cohort of children who had been seen in child guidance clinics during the 1920s. The longitudinal study (Robins 1966, 1978) examined adult outcome and showed that those who develop ASPD (or, as it was then called, "psychopathy") *always* have a prior history of conduct disorder (CD). This observation led the authors of DSM to make these antecedents a requirement for the adult disorder—a rare example in which diagnostic criteria were based on longitudinal data.

Thus, ASPD can be seen as a set of behavioral symptoms that begin in childhood and fail to remit with maturity. Most children with conduct symptoms do not develop the adult disorder; CD is a necessary but not a sufficient cause of ASPD. As noted in Chapter 1, progression to ASPD is associated with severe and early onset symptoms during childhood (Caspi 2000; Moffitt et al. 2001; Zoccolillo et al. 1996).

Borderline Personality Disorder

We know less about the precursors of borderline personality disorder (BPD). The best way to study the childhood characteristics of patients with BPD would be to conduct a prospective follow-up study of a large cohort of children, paralleling the work of Robins on ASPD.

Asking patients with BPD about their childhood does not address this issue. Most of what we *think* we know is based on long-term memories of adults about distant events. When patients with BPD describe early life experiences to therapists, the way they remember the past is strongly colored by current symptomatology. This mechanism is termed *recall bias* (Schacter 1996). When the present is going badly, perceptions of the past tend to be negative. When life goes better, perceptions become more positive. Thus, we cannot know precisely what patients were actually like as children just by taking a history.

Memories are particularly likely to be subject to recall bias in patients with BPD, in which perceptions of people and events are distorted (Paris 1995). Patients with BPD have idiosyncratic perceptions, even of *recent* life events, and are famous for seeing other people, including their therapists, as ideal or malignant (Gunderson 2001).

What childhood patterns should we look for as precursors of BPD? *CD* and *ASPD* describe similar behaviors, albeit at different ages. Yet it is not obvious that the characteristic behaviors of BPD, such as recurrent suicide attempts, severe emotional lability, or stormy intimate relationships, have clear-cut equivalents or parallels in children. Moreover, whereas CD often leads to clinical referral, few patients with BPD report having been seen by mental health care professionals prior to adolescence. In one large-scale study (Zanarini et al. 2001), the mean age at first clinical presentation was 18 years (with a standard deviation of 6 years).

On the other hand, ASPD and BPD are not as different as they seem. They have commonalities in phenomenology (Paris 1997), with symptoms that can be characterized as impulsive aggression (Coccaro et al. 1989). Risk factors such as severe family dysfunction are also similar (Paris 1997). Both disorders tend to run in the same families (Links et al. 1988; Zanarini 1993). As is shown later in this book, both have a similarly chronic course and outcome. One might therefore expect the precursors for ASPD and BPD to overlap.

Categories of disorder overlap when they share common traits. The most obvious difference between populations with ASPD and those with BPD is that patients with ASPD are usually male, whereas patients with BPD are usually female (Paris 1997). This raises the question as to whether gender influences the same traits to be expressed differently. Men are more likely to act out aggression against others, whereas women are more likely to turn aggression against themselves, differences that can be seen between boys and girls during childhood (Maccoby and Jacklin 1974).

Gender differences also suggest ways in which BPD could have different precursors from ASPD. Instead of having CD, children who later develop BPD might have a mixture of impulsive and affective symptomatology. This hypothesis is supported by a recent report from a longitudinal community study (Crawford et al. 2001a, 2001b). In general, adolescents with Cluster B symptoms tended to retain these problems in early adulthood, but externalizing symptoms predicted continuing psychopathology in boys, whereas a combination of externalizing and internalizing symptoms predicted continuing Cluster B pathology in girls.

Adult patients with BPD, about 70% of whom are female (Swartz et al. 1990), present with precisely this combination of externalizing and internalizing symptoms. They are highly impulsive, but unlike patients with ASPD, they present themselves as victims rather perpetrators. In childhood, girls develop more internalizing symptoms than boys (Achenbach and McConaughy 1997). If externalizing symptoms are less severe, and if internalizing symptoms go unnoticed, this may explain why girls at risk for BPD do not present clinically as children.

Other Cluster B Disorders

The other two categories in Cluster B, narcissistic personality disorder (NPD) and histrionic personality disorder (HPD), are less precisely defined than ASPD or BPD. (These diagnoses lack the same level of validating data.)

NPD might be understood as a less severe version of ASPD (Looper and Paris 2000). Applying Harpur et al.'s (1994) two-factor model of psychopathy, NPD shows only one of these factors: interpersonal manipulativeness, lacking the criminal behavior seen in ASPD. The close relationship between NPD and ASPD has been confirmed by a recent study (Gunderson and Ronningstam 2001). Patients from both categories showed similar characteristics on the Diagnostic Interview for Narcissism, although patients with NPD scored higher on grandiosity than did patients with ASPD.

In a parallel way, HPD could be a less severe form of BPD. It is associated with some of the same interpersonal difficulties but with much lower levels of impulsivity and affective instability. It has also been suggested (Hamburger et al. 1996) that HPD has commonalities with psychopathy but shows symptoms that reflect more typically "female" behavioral patterns.

Although one report (Nestadt et al. 1990) suggested that HPD is equally common in men, a recent community study (Torgersen et al. 2001) found

HPD to be twice as frequent in women (2.5% vs. 1.2%). In this sample, NPD had a similar prevalence (less than 1%) in both sexes. In clinical samples, men are more likely to receive a diagnosis of NPD (Carter et al. 1999). Perhaps women with narcissistic traits tend to be seen by clinicians as having HPD.

As with ASPD and BPD, NPD and HPD have some striking parallels in symptomatology, with differences related to gender. The criteria for NPD focus more on grandiosity and a need for power, classical male preoccupations, whereas those for HPD focus more on sexuality and a need to be attractive. Yet both patterns reflect an unusual need for admiration and attention. Both groups go to great lengths to obtain social reinforcements and feel crushed when these needs are not met.

We have only fragmentary data on the origins of NPD, and none at all on the origins of HPD. Behavioral genetic studies of narcissistic traits (Jang et al. 1996) and the study by Torgersen et al. (2000) of NPD and HPD all demonstrate some genetic influence. If narcissism as a trait is heritable, we should observe childhood precursors of the disorders. Guilé (2000) has identified a group of children with narcissism who have characteristics similar to those of adults with NPD. Adapting for children an instrument developed by Gunderson et al. (1990) to measure pathological narcissism in adults, Guilé found that children with narcissism, like their adult counterparts, have grandiose goals, require constant admiration, have self-esteem that is easily punctured, and suffer from rage or emptiness when the world fails to meet their needs. It would be useful to follow this cohort into adulthood, to determine the stability of these traits over time.

Finally, a large-scale community longitudinal follow-up study of children, the Albany-Saratoga study, suggests that NPD may have precursors similar to those for ASPD. Kasen et al. (2001) reported that a disruptive behavior disorder in childhood (i.e., CD and oppositional defiant disorder) increased by six times the risk for symptoms of NPD in adulthood.

Childhood Precursors of Anxious Cluster Disorders

Whereas externalizing symptoms in childhood are rooted in impulsive temperament, internalizing symptoms are rooted in anxious temperament. High levels of social anxiety can be identified as early as infancy. At the extreme, these characteristics define a syndrome of "behavioral inhibition" (Kagan 1994). When traits appear this early in development, they tend to be stable over time. Kagan has followed a cohort of behaviorally inhibited children into early adolescence, and adult outcomes will be assessed in the coming years. Early onset social anxiety in childhood may also be a precursor of anxiety disorders and/or anxious cluster personality disorders (Paris 1998a).

Anxious traits have a genetic component (Jang et al. 1996), with similar levels of heritability (close to 40%) having been documented in Cluster C personality disorders (Torgersen et al. 2000). Avoidant personality disorder and dependent personality disorder have somewhat similar symptoms (Bornstein 1997), and both disorders may derive from an anxious temperament that leads to social fearfulness, a tendency to cling to significant others, and a lack of confidence in social interactions. If Kagan's follow-up study of behaviorally inhibited children eventually shows a high prevalence of Cluster C personality disorders in adulthood, we may conclude that they are continuations of childhood patterns. Anxious traits often become problematic in adolescence, when they begin to interfere more seriously with developmental tasks. This may be more of a problem in modern societies than in traditional ones (see Chapter 1) because the former demand higher levels of individualism, with adolescents expected to plan their lives, make their own friends, and spend less time with their families.

Because anxiety and mood disorders are highly comorbid (Goldberg 2000), depression in childhood could also be a precursor of Cluster C personality disorders. Support for this hypothesis comes from the Albany-Saratoga study. Kasen et al. (2001) found that childhood depression increased the odds that symptoms of personality disorders in the C cluster would develop (14 times for the dependent category, and 10 times for the DSM-III-R category of passive-aggressive personality).

We know little about the childhood precursors of obsessive-compulsive personality disorder (OCPD). However, patients with OCPD usually describe having had similar characteristics all their lives. It seems likely that most were hard-working, unemotional, and perfectionistic as children. It would not be difficult to identify such a population, but this research has never been carried out.

All Cluster C disorders, including OCPD, are comorbid with anxiety disorders (Mavissakalian et al. 1993), but compulsive traits emerge as separate in factor analysis (Livesley et al. 1998). People with compulsive traits are not *always* anxious but experience these feelings when their world is not under control. (Unfortunately, this happens all too often.)

Gender, Symptoms, and Childhood Precursors

Externalizing symptoms are more common in boys (Achenbach and McConaughy 1997), and the most common diagnoses in children (CD, oppositional defiant disorder, attention-deficit/hyperactivity disorder), all of which are externalizing disorders, show a predominance of males (Ezpeleta et al. 2001).

In adolescence, this gender distribution changes because girls more frequently come to clinical attention as some begin to demonstrate serious impulsive behaviors (Tiet et al. 2001). Although fewer girls than boys in adolescence meet diagnostic criteria for CD, Zoccolillo et al. (1992) suggested that CD would have a more equal sex distribution if behaviors that are more deviant in females (e.g., sexual promiscuity) were given the same weighting as more typically male behaviors (e.g., physical aggression and theft). Impulsive girls are more depressed than impulsive boys, and antisocial behavior in female adolescents can precede depressive symptoms and suicide attempts (Moffitt et al. 2001). As discussed earlier, all these patterns suggest that Cluster B personality disorder symptoms in women tend to be preceded by a combination of externalizing and internalizing symptoms (Crawford et al. 2001a, 2001b).

The majority of patients in adult clinics are female, with the largest number presenting with mood and anxiety disorders (Frank 2000). Depression is two to three times more common in women than in men (Weissman and Klerman 1985). These gender differences in clinical populations most likely reflect real differences in community prevalence (Frank 2000).

Epidemiological studies find high rates of mental disorders in men that are not always seen in clinical settings (Robins and Regier 1991). For example, substance abuse and criminality are both much more common in males, with as many as 10% meeting criteria for alcoholism (Helzer and Canino 1992). Yet these men do not seek treatment to the same extent as depressed women (Robins and Regier 1991). Another well-known example of gender differences is that, whereas suicide completions are more frequent in males, suicide attempts are much more prevalent among females (Blumenthal and Kupfer 1990).

If men and women express distress though different behaviors, substance abuse and depression may not be as separate as they seem. Men could be more likely to lash out when dysphoric or to drown their sorrows in drink. Women, in contrast, seem to be more likely to express their emotions and to ask for support from others. Even in infancy, males have more difficulty with emotional regulation than do females (Weinberg et al. 1999).

These differences help explain the observation that ASPD and BPD have a "mirror-image" gender distribution. Of patients with ASPD, 80% are male (Robins and Regier 1991), whereas 70% of those meeting criteria for BPD are women (Swartz et al. 1990; Torgersen et al. 2001). Differences in overt symptoms between ASPD and BPD mask a commonality at the level of personality traits.

Personality Disorders in Childhood and Adolescence

DSM discourages the early diagnosis of personality disorders. According to the latest revision, DSM-IV-TR,

> Personality disorder categories may be applied to children and adolescents in those relatively unusual instances in which the individual's particular maladaptive personality traits appear to be pervasive, persistent, and un-likely to be limited to a particular developmental stage or an episode of an Axis I disorder. It should be recognized that the traits of a personality disorder that appear in childhood will often not persist unchanged into adult life. To diagnose a personality disorder in an individual under age 18 years, the features must have been present for at least one year. The one exception to this is antisocial personality disorder, which cannot be diagnosed in individuals under age 18 years. (p. 687)

I consider these restrictions to be mistaken and to reflect a "sentimental" prejudice. Psychiatrists have always preferred to believe that, whereas adults do not change easily, psychopathology in children and adolescents is more malleable. However, that belief is based more on emotion than on evidence. If disturbances that begin early in life have serious prognostic significance, we should be more hopeful when mental disorders present for the first time later in adulthood.

The restrictions about diagnosing ASPD are also a matter of terminology. The 17-year-old boy with severe CD is no less antisocial than he will be when he reaches his eighteenth birthday. It might make more sense to find ways to distinguish more precisely between "life-course persistent" and "adolescence-limited" antisocial behavior (Moffitt 1993), a concept that depends more on course than on symptoms. Similarly, because we know that female adolescents with disruptive behavior disorders are at high risk for personality disorders in young adulthood (Rey et al. 1997), we might see them as showing the early symptoms of Axis II pathology.

Although caution about diagnosing personality disorders in childhood is justified, a number of studies (Block et al. 1991; Garnet et al. 1994; Ludolph et al. 1990; Mattananah et al. 1995) have shown that typical cases can be identified in the adolescent years. What is confusing is that specific Axis II diagnoses do not remain stable when adolescents are followed into adulthood (Bernstein et al. 1993; Vito et al. 1999). However, diagnostic instability is not the same as recovery. Most adolescents with personality disorder symptoms continue to have serious difficulties in early adulthood (Bernstein et al. 1993). All that has happened is that behavioral patterns shift enough to move the patient from one personality disorder category to another. When patients no longer meet specific diagnostic criteria for a category, this may reflect more about the imprecision of the classification system than about the patient.

In a recent book, Paulina Kernberg et al. (2000) pointed out that we should not be misled by the difficulty of making precise diagnoses in adolescence. Personality disorders at this stage have a high level of comorbidity, which is to say that they do not form distinct patterns. Adult personality disorders are also comorbid with each other (Pfohl et al. 1986), and as we will see in later chapters, the disorders diagnosed in adults do not always remain stable on Axis II. Again, the problem lies not in the instability of the disorders but in our difficulty in classifying them.

Another caveat I have heard against diagnosing personality disorders before patients reach age 18 years is that "all adolescents are a little borderline." This point of view goes with the idea that adolescence is normally a time of turmoil and that serious disturbances at this stage can be resolved without sequelae. However, that was a misperception contradicted by the large-scale study conducted by Offer and Offer (1975) and reviewed in Chapter 1. Most adolescents in the community have a relatively smooth course to adulthood. Few are involved in delinquency or substance abuse. The majority even retain a positive view of their families.

True personality pathology in adolescence is not a transient phenomenon. In the Albany-Saratoga prospective community follow-up study (J.G. Johnson et al. 1999; Kasen et al. 1999), adolescent personality disorders predicted symptoms in young adulthood associated with Axis I disorders, Axis II disorders, substance abuse, and suicidality. Adolescents with personality disorder symptoms often have childhood histories of conduct problems, depression, and anxiety (Bernstein et al. 1993). Thus, the most prototypical cases of personality disorder involve an early onset.

In my own experience, absolutely classic cases of BPD can be seen as early as age 14. BPD, with all its classic features, has been documented in adolescent inpatients (Pinto et al. 1996) as well as outpatients (Braun-Scharm 1996). The psychosocial risk factors in these cases were also similar to those described for adults with BPD (Goldman et al. 1992; James et al. 1996).

The one point in the DSM instructions quoted above with which I do agree is that the nature of psychopathology can change over time. However, this principle applies to categories that are too fuzzy to yield more than a general continuity, whereas the trait dimensions behind personality pathology remain stable over time (Grilo et al. 2001).

This does not mean that BPD will persist into adulthood and become chronic in every instance in which it has an onset in adolescence. In my experience, personality disorders can begin in adolescence and burn out as early as age 25. A good example is provided by the following case from my follow-up study.

Ellen was a 16-year-old high school student who asked for treatment after the death by suicide of her best friend. Carla, who had been treated for BPD at the same clinic, had often talked about suicide with Ellen, who was already a chronic wrist slasher. Carla had suggested that Ellen join her in a suicide pact. Ellen declined, after which Carla jumped off a bridge.

The most unusual aspect of Ellen's clinical presentation was the variety and strength of her micropsychotic symptoms. She had intense fantasy that her life was a dream, and that she was living on another planet, where she had another existence and a real family. (Although these ideas resembled those described in Joanne Greenberg's autobiographical *I Never Promised You a Rose Garden*, Ellen was not a reader of novels.) Ellen had the belief that if she were dead, she could wake up and return to her true home on the other planet. She would hear the voices of individual characters in this fantasy speaking to her and asking her to join them.

Ellen had a very traumatic history. At age 16, she was living with her older sister, after running away first from both her alcoholic mother and then from a strongly paranoid father who had incestuously abused her. She had even made a first suicide attempt at age 10, leaping from a first-story balcony after a quarrel with her mother. This episode led to Ellen's first clinical presentation, in a child psychiatry clinic.

Ellen was accepted into weekly outpatient psychotherapy, and she attended regularly for the next 2 years. Her treatment course was punctuated by several overdoses of medication, which led to medical hospitalizations. She also continued to self-mutilate, on one occasion carving my name onto her arm. She also continue to be obsessed with Carla. On the anniversary of Carla's death, she expressed a strong wish to join her and indicated that she could not control this impulse.

Ellen's subsequent hospitalization lasted a month. Admission carried the patient past the ominous anniversary. Family therapy helped support her sister and brother-in-law in caring for her and also helped Ellen keep her distance from her mother and father. Finally, Ellen was given trifluoperazine, which controlled her psychotic symptoms over the next few months.

Ellen remained in psychotherapy from age 16 to age 19. She made impressive gains during this time, shedding both her suicidality and her psychotic symptomatology. When she was given follow-up evaluations, first at age 25 and then at age 38, she had no symptoms of BPD.

I have documented Ellen's symptoms in some detail to demonstrate the classic nature of her clinical picture, which met all the criteria for BPD. Nonetheless, she made an early, complete, and stable recovery (described in Chapter 8). Although chronicity is the rule for personality disorders, individual patients can vary in their course. Ellen, and others like her, can have all the features of BPD early in life and still recover. Patients whose disorders remit early should not be automatically considered as having another illness. Medical illnesses also vary in prognosis. Even the most chronic diseases, such as rheumatoid arthritis, bronchial asthma, or multiple sclerosis show variable courses. Some patients recover remarkably, whereas others deteriorate. It will take more time and more research on the causes of these illnesses to find out why.

Future Research Strategies

The relationship between personality disorders and their precursors is not linear. Although temperamental factors can be precursors of pathology, among children with difficult temperaments, only a minority develop disorders (Lykken 1995). Childhood adversities can be precursors of pathology, but among children who suffer psychological and social disadvantage, most remain resilient (Rutter 1987a; Werner and Smith 1992).

The most reliable source of information on how early experience shapes adult life must come from prospective longitudinal studies of children in community populations. This strategy can also address the problem of whether continuities reflect temperament or experience.

There have been only a relatively small number of investigations of this kind. (For reviews, see Kagan and Zentner 1996; Paris 2000c.) Such studies are expensive and time-consuming. They also demand faith from funding agencies, as well as determination from investigators with a reasonably long life expectancy.

Some investigations have begun their follow-up evaluations in infancy. The earliest and best-known project was the New York Longitudinal Study (Chess and Thomas 1984), which followed a group of normal children from infancy to early adulthood. This study showed that having a "difficult" temperament is associated with poorer functioning in young adulthood. However, the Chess and Thomas sample was small, and it lacked a wide range of variability. For this reason, later research has focused on temperamental extremes, following samples at greater risk. One good example is Kagan's (1994) follow-up study of behaviorally inhibited infants. Another is the follow-up study by Caspi et al. (1996) of a birth cohort in which undercontrolled and inhibited behavior at age 3 years were predictors of, respectively, antisocial personality and depression at age 21 years.

Temperament should be measured in early childhood. However, temperamental patterns have been shown to become stable by age 2 years (Rothbart et al. 2000). If we were to start at this stage, we could be relatively sure that we were looking at inborn characteristics rather than effects of life stressors. The earlier in development temperamental precursors appear, the more likely they should be to persist over time and lead to psychopathology.

Other follow-up studies have begun follow-up evaluation somewhat later in development, using childhood behaviors as predictors of adult symptoms. In one of the largest-scale investigations, Tremblay et al. (1994) conducted a longitudinal study of a community sample from age 6 onward. The results concerning adult outcome are still coming in, but one early finding has confirmed that externalizing symptoms during middle childhood are predictive of delinquency and substance abuse during adolescence (Masse and Tremblay 1997).

Another research project of this kind has been led by Pat Cohen of Columbia University. At previously discussed, this is a long-term follow-up study of a community cohort of children in the Albany-Saratoga area of New York State. This is one of the very few studies that has used personality disorder as an outcome variable. However, because few cases met formal diagnostic criteria, instead of measuring the categorical presence or absence of personality disorder, the researchers created a scale by counting the number of symptoms in each category. This method yielded results that otherwise might not have emerged. For example, the researchers were able to show that psychosocial adversities during childhood (trauma and neglect) predicted personality disorder symptoms in young adulthood (J.G. Johnson et al. 1999).

Another research strategy would involve the identification of biological correlates and markers for temperamental variations. These markers might consist of genotypes or changes in neurotransmitter activity (Siever et al. 1998). My own group is presently conducting such a study, using a large community sample from Quebec that has been studied by Richard Tremblay at the University of Montreal. Studies of this type will also help to provide more precise answers about the precursors of personality disorders.

With unlimited funds and ready access to community populations, one might imagine an ideal prospective strategy. This could involve

- Recruiting a large enough sample to study multiple variables
- Factoring out the role of genetics in personality development by following a large sample of identical and fraternal twins
- Genotyping subjects
- Studying children from infancy onward, for a baseline of temperament
- Making regular assessments of parenting behavior over the course of childhood
- Measuring the influence of factors outside the family (social class, quality of schools, peer groups, community)
- Applying multiple measures of outcome: behavior, symptoms, functioning, diagnoses, and traits

Although such a project seems like a very formidable undertaking, a research group in Canada (under Daniel Pérusse at the University of Montreal) is presently conducting a study precisely along these lines. The investigators are collecting data on hundreds of twins whose environment and development will be examined regularly over time and then followed into adulthood. This study is specifically designed to determine the temperamental and environmental precursors of personality disorders.

Although the ideal way to determine the childhood precursors of mental disorders involves prospective research on community samples of children, this method is most useful for high-prevalence disorders. For example, mood disorders, anxiety disorders, and alcoholism, all with lifetime prevalence rates ranging up to 10%, are particularly suitable, but for disorders such as schizophrenia and bipolar illness, each of which has a prevalence of about 1%, or for ASPD or BPD, with prevalences in the same range, community samples will not yield enough patients with diagnosable disorders. Even with a sample of 1,000, one might find only 10–20 individuals with the index pathology. (This is what happened in the Albany-Saratoga study.)

An alternative way to address this problem would be to study high-risk populations. By identifying groups of children at biological and/or psychosocial risk and then following them prospectively, we maximize our chances of identifying patients with disorders. This strategy has its own limitation, in that high-risk populations may not be representative of those who eventually develop the disorder under study. Nonetheless, Chapter 3 examines how this method can be used to examine precursors of Cluster B personality disorder.

3

Borderline Pathology of Childhood

This chapter describes two high-risk strategies to identify precursors for Cluster B personality disorders. The first is to study a group of children whose disorders have been labeled "borderline." The second is to examine the children of parents with borderline personality disorder (BPD).

Which children are most at risk for personality disorders, and why? One factor could be an abnormal temperament. Another is that children likely to develop disorders later in life have been subjected to severe and multiple adversities, whose cumulative effects produce psychopathology (Rutter and Rutter 1993). Both patterns would be more likely to be found in a high-risk group.

Measuring biological vulnerability in children could help to determine the causes of personality disorders. We also need to study children who *recently* experienced life adversities. In retrospective studies, adult patients with BPD tend to report trauma and/or neglect during childhood (Zanarini 2000). Yet community studies (Browne and Finkelhor 1986; Rind and Tromovitch 1997; Rind et al. 1998) show that most children exposed to these adversities do not develop serious psychopathology. Direct examination of the impact of life events on vulnerable children can help sort out these pathways to psychopathology.

Defining Borderline Pathology of Childhood

There is a group of children whose pathology has long been described in the literature as "borderline" (Kernberg 1991), largely because their clinical symptoms resemble adult BPD. These children have histories of trauma and neglect (Goldman et al. 1992) that resemble the adversities described by adult patients. Studying this population could be a first step toward understanding the precursors of Cluster B personality disorders.

The term *borderline pathology of childhood* describes a complex and severe behavioral syndrome seen in latency-aged children (Greenman et al. 1986; Kernberg 1991). The clinical picture is characterized by a mixture of pathology on several dimensions—externalizing, internalizing, and cognitive. These children are highly impulsive but may also be suicidally depressed and/or have micropsychotic symptoms. Thus, these children resemble adults with BPD and may have similar temperamental characteristics.

The use of the term *borderline* for this population makes sense only in a historical context. Borderline personality in adult patients is also a misnomer (Paris 1994), reflecting older concepts that all psychopathology lies on a continuum and that patients can live on a "border" between neurosis and psychosis. However, the presence of behavioral disorganization and micropsychotic features in children has led several observers (Bemporad and Ciccheti 1982; Robson 1983) to suggest that this condition lies on the same border as BPD.

What are children with borderline pathology like? Unlike adult patients with BPD, but like most children seen in psychiatry, the majority are boys. To illustrate their clinical presentation, I describe here a typical example.

Carlos, a 9-year-old boy, was referred to a child psychiatry clinic after being expelled from school for disruptive behavior in class. When confronted by the school principal after one of these incidents, he threatened to jump out of the window.

Carlos was described by both his family and his teachers as an angry and unhappy child. He had no friends and never enjoyed activities such as sports or games. His mother stated that he had always been difficult and overly sensitive. In recent months, he had several times told her he wished he was dead. He would fall into rages in which he would sometimes bang his head against walls. Carlos had been close to failing in school for the past year. At home, his behavior varied from demanding and clinging to argumentative and hostile.

Carlos's father, an alcoholic man who had left the mother quite early on, had since played no role in child care. The mother was a chronically depressed woman who had been a client of several social agencies and had also been seen in psychiatric consultation. Carlos had lived in a foster home between the ages of 3 and 5 years, until his mother reclaimed him.

On examination, Carlos was a sad and withdrawn child. He had a vague manner and described himself as "spaced out." After being drawn out, he described a vivid and intense fantasy life. In particular, he sometimes believed himself to be in contact with a foster brother, James, whom he had not seen in 4 years. He regularly heard James's voice in his head talking to him, although he was not actually sure whether this was his imagination.

Carlos's symptoms demonstrate some of the reasons why the term *borderline* has been applied to this population. The clinical picture shows a number of symptomatic resemblances to BPD in adults, which also includes a combination of impulsive, affective, and cognitive features. Carlos's history also demonstrates the mixture of trauma and neglect common in these patients.

The earliest descriptions of borderline pathology in children (Bemporad and Ciccheti 1982; Kestenbaum 1983; Pine 1974) were based on clinical observation rather than on systematic criteria. For this reason, children with borderline pathology have been a heterogeneous population (Petti and Vela 1990). Later, more precise criteria were developed (Goldman et al. 1992; Greenman et al. 1986), focusing on childhood behaviors that specifically parallel symptoms seen in adult BPD.

Borderline pathology of childhood should not be thought of as an earlier version of the adult category. It is just as likely to be a unique syndrome. Some researchers (Cohen et al. 1987; Lincoln et al. 1998) have suggested avoiding the term *borderline* entirely, replacing it with the more neutral and descriptive construct of *multiple complex developmental disorder.* This terminology emphasizes the presence of multiple symptom dimensions in these patients (Ad-Dab'bagh and Greenfield 2001). This symptomatic complexity makes it more likely that borderline pathology of childhood, even more than other precursors of adult pathology (such as conduct disorder and attention-deficit/hyperactivity disorder), will lead to long-term sequelae.

Children with borderline pathology do not necessarily turn into adults with BPD. Thus far, only one follow-up study has specifically addressed their long-term outcome. Lofgren et al. (1991) followed a small cohort (19 children) who had met a set of criteria for borderline pathology developed by Bemporad and Ciccheti (1982). These children developed a wide range of Axis II disorders by age 18 years and did not have Axis I diagnoses such as schizophrenia or bipolar mood disorder.

Thus, borderline pathology in childhood could be a precursor for a wide range of adult personality disorders. Given the prominent impulsive symptoms, one might have expected this group to be at particular risk for developing Cluster B disorders. Yet the Axis II diagnoses in the cohort studied by Lofgren et al. fell into all three clusters, with no particular predominance for BPD. It is possible that these findings are an artifact of the criteria used—that is, that the outcome was heterogeneous because the original cohort was heterogeneous. These findings must be replicated in a larger sample, and future research must use more precise methods for establishing a baseline diagnosis.

In another study of a similar cohort, Kumra et al. (1998) examined 19 children referred for atypical psychotic symptoms who were eventually diagnosed as having "multidimensionally impaired disorder." These children had, in addition to micropsychotic symptoms, daily periods of emotional lability, impaired interpersonal skills, and cognitive deficits in information processing. Although Kumra et al. referred to the similar concepts of Cohen et al. (1987) on *multiple complex developmental disorder*, they did not use the term *borderline* to describe these children. Instead, they suggested that the children might have a disorder in the schizophrenic spectrum. However, when 26 children with this clinical picture were reevaluated at a mean age of 15 years (2–8 years after the original evaluation [Nicolson et al. 2001]), most showed remission of psychotic symptoms, and many developed features of a chronic mood disorder. Although these researchers never used the term *borderline* (and never made Axis II diagnoses for these adolescents), it seems likely that they were looking at the same kind of patients.

The psychosocial risk factors associated with borderline pathology of childhood and adulthood are strikingly similar to those described by adults with BPD. The early clinical literature had suggested that these children often come from dysfunctional families characterized by trauma, neglect, and separation (Bemporad and Ciccheti 1982; Kestenbaum 1983). These observations have been supported by systematic empirical findings that sexual and physical abuse are common among children and adolescents with borderline pathology (Goldman et al. 1992, 1993). The parents of children with borderline pathology also have serious psychopathology, often disorders in the impulsive spectrum (Feldman et al. 1995; Goldman et al. 1992, 1993; Weiss et al. 1996). This finding is important because, in contrast to retrospective reports from adult patients, direct observations in children avoid recall bias and can be validated by family members and health professionals.

Borderline pathology of childhood has been associated with neuropsychological abnormalities. The findings include "soft" signs of organicity, such as learning disabilities, attention-deficit/hyperactivity disorder, and abnormal electroencephalogram patterns (Lincoln et al. 1998; Petti and Vela 1990). These symptoms are not specific to children with borderline pathology, because they are seen in a wide range of behavioral disorders. It is also not clear whether these neuropsychological abnormalities are constitutional or environmental in origin. For example, similar symptoms are seen in children with posttraumatic stress disorder (Beers and De Bellis 2002), raising the question of whether life events affect brain circuitry. Nonetheless, research confirms a robust relationship between deficits in the ability to plan ahead, termed *executive functioning*, and impulsive personality traits (Stein et al. 1993). These neuropsychological findings, which point to abnormalities in the prefrontal cortex, are seen in most disorders characterized by impulsivity, including adult BPD (O'Leary 2000).

The Montreal Research Project on Children with Borderline Pathology

Our research group (Jaswant Guzder, Phyllis Zelkowitz, Ron Feldman, and I) has been carrying out a systematic study of borderline pathology in children. The first step involved a chart review for a cohort of 98 children (79 boys and 19 girls) in day treatment (Guzder et al. 1996). Using a structured instrument specifically designed to identify borderline pathology, the Child Version of the Retrospective Diagnostic Interview for Borderlines (C-DIB-R [Greenman et al. 1986]), we divided the sample into a group of 41 meeting research criteria and a group of 57 who did not. Notably, over 40% of children in day treatment met these criteria, pointing to the clinical importance of studying this group.

We set the bar high by using a comparison group that was also sick enough to require day treatment. All of our patients had been referred because their condition could not be managed in the school system, and all had low levels of global functioning. However, in comparing the two groups, we made sure that any findings specific to borderline pathology were independent of severity of impairment. In addition, we measured a number of comorbid diagnoses, most particularly conduct disorder, that were equally frequent in both groups and that did not account for differences between them.

We found several adversities to be more common in the children with borderline pathology, including sexual abuse, physical abuse, and extreme neglect. At the same time, children with borderline pathology were more likely to have parents with histories of substance abuse and criminality. In multivariate analyses, sexual abuse and extreme neglect emerged as independent predictors of diagnosis, as did scales measuring the cumulative effects of multiple risks (particularly abuse and parental dysfunction).

The next step of our research program was to conduct a more detailed cross-sectional study. We examined a separate cohort of 94 children (81 boys and 13 girls) attending the same child psychiatry day treatment center, this time using direct assessment instead of chart review. To establish the diagnosis, we used the same instrument (C-DIB-R); again, 40% of the sample met criteria. We also developed an index to measure psychosocial stressors (drawn from clinical observations by multiple therapists during the time the children were in the unit).

The results confirmed the chart review findings (Guzder et al. 1999). Children with borderline pathology, compared with those without it, had an increased frequency of parental neglect and childhood sexual abuse. Again, the group with borderline pathology was significantly more likely to have parents with histories of substance abuse and criminality. Although conduct disorder was significantly more common in the group with borderline pathology, comorbidity did not account for differences in risk factors.

The cross-sectional study added measures of neuropsychological functioning. A standard battery showed several significant differences between the two groups, most particularly on the Continuous Performance Test and the Wisconsin Card Sorting Test (Paris et al. 1999). Compared with other children undergoing day treatment, those with borderline pathology had more difficulty with attention, control of impulses, and concept formation. These findings pointed to defective executive function. Finally, we were able to show that the neuropsychological and psychosocial risk factors made independent contributions to the discrimination between children with borderline pathology and those without it (Zelkowitz et al. 2001).

The neuropsychological findings of our work are of theoretical interest. Applying a stress–diathesis model (Monroe and Simons 1991; Paris 1999) to borderline pathology of childhood, we believe these children to have a combination of temperamental vulnerability and stressful adversities. Our methods could not fully separate the effects of temperament and life experience. Although it is possible that life events cause neuropsychological abnormalities, children with borderline pathology could have inborn abnormalities in brain "wiring." Psychosocial risk factors would act as environmental stressors, unleashing these diatheses.

The important issue not yet addressed by our program is long-term outcome. The next step will require reassessment of the cohort as they reach adolescence and then as they reach young adulthood. We are presently carrying out this study. Thus far, we have data on a subgroup ($n=35$) of our original cohort, at a mean age of 15 years. These preliminary results (Zelkowitz et al. 2001) indicate that children with borderline pathology continue to function at a low level during adolescence, worse than other graduates of our day program.

Children of Borderline Parents

The second high-risk strategy we used for determining precursors of BPD involved studying children whose parents had this disorder. It is well established (Zanarini 1993) that patients with BPD tend to have relatives who also have disorders in the impulsive spectrum (i.e., substance abuse, antisocial personality disorder, and sometimes but not necessarily, BPD itself). Several studies (Johnson et al. 1995; Links et al. 1988; Riso et al. 2000) have involved direct interviewing of family members of patients with borderline pathology. Although each of these reports found increased rates of personality disorders, including BPD, in first-degree relatives of probands, they also observed higher rates for mood disorders and impulsive spectrum disorders. It would therefore be of some interest to determine whether the *children* of parents with BPD are at risk for the same disorder or for similar disorders.

Our research group had collected a sample of 78 women with BPD for a large-scale study of BPD in adulthood (Paris et al. 1994a). As Stone (1990) documented, and as was later confirmed in our own follow-up studies (Paris and Zweig-Frank 2001), the women with BPD tend to have few children. Thus, only 9 members of this cohort had become mothers by a mean age of 30 years.

These women were raising a total of 21 children ranging in age from latency to adolescence. We compared their offspring with a sample of 21 children whose mothers had other nonborderline personality disorders (and who had served as control subjects in our original study). The findings (Weiss et al. 1996) showed that the children of mothers with BPD, compared with control subjects, had significantly more psychiatric diagnoses, more impulse control disorders, a higher frequency of borderline pathology of childhood (as measured by the C-DIB-R), and lower scores on the Children's Global Assessment Scale. In a separate report (Feldman et al. 1995), we compared family structure in these two groups using the Family Environment Scale (Moos 1990) and found that families with mothers who had BPD had significantly lower levels of cohesion.

These results suggest that having a mother with BPD constitutes a major risk factor for psychopathology in children. The findings were even more striking given that the comparison group also had mothers with personality disorders. In fact, rates of psychopathology and levels of family dysfunction were so high in both groups that we concluded that having a parent with *any* Axis II disorder constitutes a significant risk.

Common genetic vulnerabilities could be one factor in this association. Parents with extreme temperaments should be more likely to have children with similar problems, but the environment in these families was also very disturbed. Moreover, the family problems associated with Axis II diagnoses in parents are *continuous* (rather than episodic, as in mood disorders). In support of this interpretation, Rutter and Quinton (1984) found the effects of parental personality disorders on children to be generally more severe than parental Axis I pathology.

Conclusions

These studies of high-risk populations do not provide definitive answers about the precursors of Cluster B personality disorders. We need to monitor both cohorts to determine the extent to which symptoms continue into adulthood. Even without knowing the ultimate outcome of their pathology, we can state with assurance that these groups of children will need high levels of care from psychiatry clinics.

However, the results of these studies cannot be readily generalized to adult patients with BPD. Whereas most children with borderline pathology are male, most adults with it are female. Mental health care professionals are missing troubled girls, who can be "invisible" at this stage unless their home situation is bad enough to require legal intervention. Our study would have had a more equal distribution of boys and girls if we had studied borderline pathology in adolescence, when girls come to attention through symptoms such as shoplifting, running away from home, or sexual promiscuity. However, it is much more difficult to measure childhood adversities in girls of that age. In addition, some women with BPD, in spite of having been exposed to grave childhood adversities, do not develop serious problems until early adulthood. Similarly, the results of the study of children with parents who have BPD are not generalizable to most patients who develop BPD. Only a minority have mothers with the same pathology, and as Links et al. (1988) found, some of these patients do not have a first-degree relative with an externalizing disorder.

Ultimately, we hope to study a population of children in which adversities such as trauma and neglect are common, and then follow them prospectively over time. We are currently planning to study a cohort referred to a child protection agency because of abuse and neglect. This approach could determine more precisely the extent to which at-risk children are vulnerable to personality disorders in adulthood. This research plan faces practical problems, because considerations of privacy make it difficult to identify children at risk and to follow them prospectively. It is ethically problematic to conduct long-term studies of abused children whose identity is protected under the law. Nonetheless, previous researchers have obtained and used court data to identify these populations (and to confirm that they were in fact traumatized) and have gone on to follow them as adults. The best study (Widom 1999) confirmed that abused and neglected children are at much higher risk for adult psychopathology.

In spite of these limitations, our work offers a few clues to the larger puzzle. Children at risk for personality disorders have early onset symptoms that may reflect temperamental vulnerability and/or defective brain "wiring." At the same time, these are children exposed to highly adverse environments. This combination of biological and psychosocial risks could be particularly likely to amplify traits into disorders. This model of gene–environment interaction is applied in Chapter 4 to a general theory of personality disorders that can account for their course in adulthood.

4

Personality Disorders in Adulthood

In this chapter, I present a general theoretical model of personality disorders. I suggest that these conditions can be understood as pathological exaggerations of traits that become amplified through interactions between genetic predispositions, psychological stressors, and social factors. I show how this model helps account for their origins and for their chronic course during adulthood. I illustrate the theory with data on specific Axis II categories.

Temperament, Traits, and Personality Disorders

Temperament, traits, and disorders lie in a *hierarchy*, each "nested" in the next level (Rutter 1987b; see Figure 4–1). *Temperament* refers to inborn tendencies that shape behavior, thought, and emotion; individual differences in temperament have a genetic basis (Rothbart et al. 2000).

Personality traits are stable characteristics affecting behavior, emotion, and thought that differ between individuals. Traits derive from an amalgam of temperament and experience (Rutter 1989) and have a wide range of normal variation. Ultimately, traits are adaptations to different environmental challenges (Beck and Freeman 1990).

Personality disorders are diagnosed when traits cause dysfunction. Thus, there is no clear cutoff point between traits and disorders (Livesley et al. 1998), but disorders tend to be associated with unusual or extreme personality traits, which are, in turn, rooted in temperament (Kagan 1994). Trait amplification is also mediated by exposure to psychological and social stressors (Rutter 1987b).

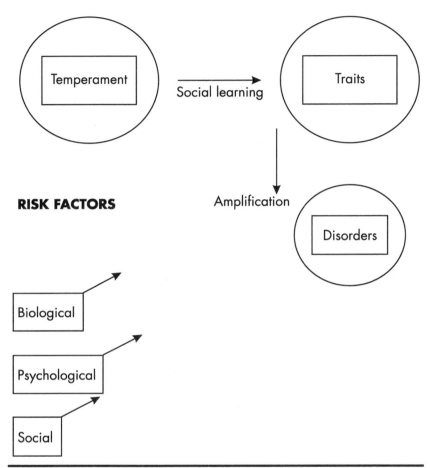

FIGURE 4–1.   Personality: temperament, traits, and disorders.

Genetic Factors in Personality Disorders

Personality is heritable. A wide range of behavioral genetic studies (reviewed in Plomin et al. 2000), based on twin and adoption studies, have shown that about half the variance in personality traits can be accounted for by genetic differences.

Because disorders are continuous with traits, one would expect them to have similar levels of heritability. Some theorists (e.g., Nigg and Goldsmith 1994) have suggested that personality disorders could be less heritable than traits, with environmental factors being more important. This has not turned out to be the case. The large twin series from Norway studied by Torgersen et al. (2000) showed conclusively that personality disorders have a genetic component quite similar to that influencing trait dimensions. The heritability coefficient was 0.60 for Axis II disorders as a whole, 0.37 for Cluster A, 0.60 for Cluster B, and 0.62 for Cluster C. In borderline personality disorder (BPD), often thought to be mainly the result of childhood adversity, heritable factors accounted for as much as 69% of the variance.

The study by Torgersen et al. is the most extensive behavioral genetic research ever conducted on personality disorders. The main caveat to keep in mind is that heritability coefficients depend on the characteristics of the sample. Torgersen et al. attributed the lower heritability in the A cluster to a higher base rate in the Norwegian population, the effect of cultural factors within a traditionally rural and isolated society.

These findings should not be interpreted as showing that there are genes "for" personality disorder. Diseases are heritable, but that is not what genes do. DNA makes proteins, which indirectly affects behavior. Moreover, because the inheritance of complex traits is affected by many alleles, variations in any single gene account for only a small percentage of the variance. If, for example, 20 or 25 genes, in various combinations, were to affect traits of impulsivity, while another 20 or 25 (not necessarily the same ones) were to influence affective instability, the complexity of these relationships would be enormous.

The findings of research also depend on how we measure personality traits. Most research instruments derive from factor analysis of questionnaire data, but this method provides only a rough guide to personality. Once the neural mechanisms behind traits are known, these dimensions will probably be redefined on a biological basis (Jang et al. 2001; Paris 2000b). In the meantime, we must make do with what we have.

Personality schema can describe "narrow" or "broad" dimensions. Narrow dimensions are a large number of specific behavioral clusters, whereas broad dimensions are a smaller number of characteristics. Owing to their simplicity, broad schema have been more popular.

The five-factor model (Costa and McCrae 1988) has been widely used in research. It describes traits of extraversion, neuroticism, openness to experience, conscientiousness, and agreeableness. The Temperament and Character Inventory (Cloninger et al. 1993; Svrakic et al. 1993) is another popular instrument that describes temperamental dimensions of novelty seeking, reward dependence, harm avoidance, and persistence (as well as three dimensions of "character"). Still another schema derives from an instrument developed by Canadian psychiatrist John Livesley, whose factor analysis of 18 narrow dimensions also yielded broader traits: emotional dysregulation, dissocial behavior, inhibitedness, and compulsivity (Livesley et al. 1998). All these competing schema are rather similar, with the same characteristics ending up clustering together (Clark and Livesley 2002).

Because broad personality dimensions describe highly complex phenomena, traits lack strong or consistent relationships with specific genes

(Livesley, in press). Research findings in this area have certainly been inconsistent. Benjamin et al. (1996) found a relationship between scores for novelty seeking and changes at an allele (DRD4) involved in dopamine metabolism, but the gene accounted for only a small percent of the variance. Lesch et al. (1996) found a link between neuroticism and variations in an allele related to the serotonin transporter. (These results even made their way into an issue of *Time* magazine. Unfortunately, the fact that other groups failed to replicate the original finding was never discussed by the popular media.)

Genetic variations associated with traits can also be associated with biological markers, which may be neurochemical, neurophysiological, or neuropsychological (Mann 1998; Siever and Davis 1991). These correlates of personality disorders are discussed below in relation to specific categories on Axis II.

Gene–Environment Interactions in Personality Disorders

Behavioral genetics sheds light on the environmental component in personality. Although half of the variance in traits (Plomin et al. 2000) and half of the variance in disorders (Torgersen et al. 2000) derive from nongenetic factors, these effects all come from the "unshared environment"—that is, from experiences unique to the individual.

I was taught that disorders that begin early in life must be the result of even earlier adversities, and that the earlier an adversity occurs, the more disruption in personality structure it will cause. Personality pathology was seen as the outcome of defective parenting, from infancy onward. However, the lack of shared environmental effects on personality challenges traditional ideas. The only way to reconcile these findings with classical theory would be to assume that environmental effects are unshared because parents treat their children differently. However, research indicates that parents tend to raise children similarly and that what differences occur are in response to the child's temperament (Reiss et al. 2000).

Gathering evidence supports a more nuanced approach. Patients with personality disorders (particularly in the antisocial and borderline categories) tend to have a history of childhood adversity and family dysfunction. Yet most children exposed to these experiences never develop serious psychopathology (Rutter 1987a). This observation applies even to serious trauma such as childhood sexual abuse (Browne and Finkelhor 1986; Rind and Tromovitch 1997; Rind et al. 1998). Moreover, studies of the siblings of personality disorder patients (Links et al. 1988) show them to be at higher risk for psychopathology, but they do not necessarily develop the same disorder—or, for that matter, any disorder. This supports the conclusion that adverse experiences during childhood cannot, by themselves, account for the origins of personality disorders.

The most likely answer to this problem is that personality develops through gene–environment interactions and that personality disorders are the results of interactions between predispositions and stressors. The effects of adversity are greater in individuals who are predisposed to psychopathology (Rutter and Rutter 1993). Although childhood trauma increases the overall risk for pathology, these relationships are largely accounted for by vulnerable subpopulations (Paris 1996). Children who develop personality disorders probably begin life with an abnormal temperament.

Temperamental abnormalities are associated with a greater sensitivity to environmental risk factors, more traumatic events, and more negative interactions with other people (Rutter and Maughan 1997). Children with high levels of aggression and irritability are often in chronic conflict with parents, peers, and teachers but may respond to these conflicts with even greater aggression (Rutter and Quinton 1984). Similarly, children with behavioral inhibition elicit overprotective responses, which only makes the problem worse (Kagan 1994). These feedback loops can spiral out of control, exaggerating existing traits, making them difficult to change later in life. Finally, the more adversities a child experiences, the greater are the cumulative effects (Rutter and Rutter 1993).

In summary, this model sees personality disorders as emerging from interactions between temperamental vulnerability and the cumulative effects of multiple psychosocial adversities. The model also suggests that predispositions unique to each individual determine what type of disorder will develop. These gene–environment interactions do not stop when children reach adulthood. Negative feedback loops between problematic traits and stressful life experiences continue to shape the course of personality disorders and help account for their chronicity.

Applying the Model to Specific Categories of Disorder

I now apply the general model of personality disorders to specific categories. I focus on four of these (antisocial, borderline, narcissistic, and avoidant), which have the largest empirical and clinical literatures. In each case, I discuss biological, psychological, and social factors in etiology and outline some clinical implications of the model. Finally, I discuss, more briefly, what is known about the other categories on Axis II.

Antisocial Personality Disorder

Antisocial personality disorder (ASPD) describes individuals whose behavior runs consistently against social norms. These individuals have not always been seen as ill (Berrios 1993). A turning point came when Cleckley (1964) described a mental illness called "psychopathy," characterized by abnormal relationships and serious deficits in empathy. The DSM definition of ASPD uses a somewhat narrower concept, which emphasizes irresponsibility and criminality. Harpur et al. (1994), who developed a widely used instrument to measure the older construct of psychopathy, criticized DSM for failing to give proper weight to abnormalities in interpersonal relationships. However, because psychopathy and ASPD are closely related, I examine here research using either construct.

Biological Factors

Owing to their lack of cooperativeness with research, we have little twin data on patients with ASPD. The study of twins conducted by Torgersen et al. (2000) recruited no subjects at all in this category. It has been shown that antisocial traits such as impulsivity and risk-taking are heritable (Plomin et al. 1990). Moreover, adoption studies (Cloninger et al. 1982; Mednick et al. 1984) show that children of parents with ASPD tend to develop similar behaviors, even in normal families.

Patients with ASPD have consistent abnormalities on neuropsychological testing, with defects in executive function and planning related to the prefrontal cortex (Sutker et al. 1993). Raine et al. (2001) reported structural changes in the brain in patients with ASPD, with a decrease in prefrontal gray matter, which could be related to differences in executive function. Patients with ASPD also fail to develop conditioned responses to fear (Harpur et al. 1994; Mednick et al. 1984). These observations mesh well with theories of psychopathy (Cleckley 1964; Eysenck 1977) that suggest that these patients lack normal anxiety, leading to a failure to learn from negative experiences. This could be why individuals with ASPD who are in the military sometimes function well in combat, even becoming heroes, yet end up in prison during peacetime (Yochelson and Samenow 1976).

Kagan (1994) labeled the constitutional factor in antisocial personality "uninhibited temperament" (in contrast to the inhibited temperament of a shy child). Kagan argued that being temperamentally outgoing and active is not sufficient by itself to cause criminality but is a necessary precondition for its development. In contrast, an inhibited temperament would be strongly protective *against* criminality. Thus, uninhibited temperament in childhood would be associated with externalizing symptoms such as conduct disorder

(CD) and hyperactivity. CD is the defined precursor for ASPD, and about one-third of hyperactive children develop antisocial behavior in adolescence and young adulthood (Weiss and Hechtman 1993; West and Farrington 1973). Thus, antisocial personality is clearly rooted in preexisting traits.

Using the five-factor model, the personality dimensions underlying the disorder have been hypothesized to include low neuroticism, low agreeableness, and low conscientiousness (Costa and Widiger 1994). Research (e.g., Hart and Hare 1994) has generally confirmed these relationships. Using the Temperament and Character Inventory, the trait profile of ASPD would be described as high novelty-seeking, low reward dependence, and low harm avoidance (Cloninger 1987).

Using a model based on variations in neurotransmitter activity, Siever and Davis (1991) proposed that ASPD derives from two temperamental abnormalities: impulsivity (modulated by low levels of serotonin) and increased behavioral activation (modulated by high levels of monoamines). Although this hypothesis has not been exhaustively studied, men with the trait of "impulsive aggression" are established to have sluggish central serotonin activity (Coccaro et al. 1989).

Any theory of ASPD must account for the fact that most patients who have it are male (Robins and Regier 1991). The gender difference is real, but it also reflects how men and women express pathology derived from similar traits through different behavioral patterns; from childhood on, males have higher levels of physical aggression (Maccoby and Jacklin 1974).

Psychological Factors

The most consistent finding concerning psychological risks in ASPD is that these patients tend to come from dysfunctional families in which discipline is inconsistent, varying unpredictably between excessive punishment and noninvolvement (Lykken 1995; Robins 1966). Parental psychopathology is common in these families, whereas abuse and neglect are ubiquitous (Rutter and Smith 1995).

There can be no doubt that antisocial children are exposed to severe adversities in childhood. However, the effects of these adversities depend on interactions with temperamental factors: These children have impulsive responses to dysphoria and deal with stressful situations by acting out, behaviors that often lead to even more mistreatment (Lykken 1995).

Social Factors

ASPD was the only personality disorder included in two large-scale American surveys of mental illness: the Epidemiological Catchment Area (ECA) study (Robins and Regier 1991) and the National Comorbidity Survey

(NCS; Kessler et al. 1994). Its prevalence was found to be similar in several English-speaking countries, with rates ranging between 2.4% and 3.7% (see review in Paris 1996). A recent study from the ECA in Baltimore (Samuels et al. 2002) yielded a figure as high as 5%. Antisocial behavior is far more common in young people, in males, and in the lower socioeconomic classes, but ASPD does not show differential prevalence by race, and there are no differences between ethnic groups living in the same American cities (Robins and Regier 1991).

Poverty does not explain antisocial behavior. The greatest increase in the prevalence of criminality took place in Western countries in the decades following World War II, in the face of unprecedented prosperity (Rutter and Rutter 1993). Robins (1966) found that relationships between lower socioeconomic status and antisocial behavior are not independent of criminality in fathers. Thus, poverty does not lead to crime when families are functioning well. Snarey and Vaillant (1985), in a long-term follow-up study of an inner-city sample of young males, found that most people raised in slums work hard to make their lives better and never turn to crime.

Historically, these relationships may have been different. Two hundred years ago, Great Britain exiled large numbers of "criminals" to Australia (Hughes 1988). Most were involved in petty offenses such as stealing. These behaviors were related to levels of poverty that would not be tolerated in modern society. The culture that developed in the new country provided many opportunities for the descendants of the original settlers. Today, Australia is a prosperous country, with a crime rate no higher than that for the British Isles.

In modern society, social structures are more important than economics in generating antisocial behavior. ASPD has shown dramatic increases in prevalence in North America, doubling among young people in the decades after World War II (Kessler et al. 1994; Robins and Regier 1991). Social change must be responsible for these cohort effects. The post-war world in the West was marked by the breakdown of social networks, as well as by increases in family dissolution, unbuffered by traditional sources of social support, such as extended family and community.

The most powerful evidence for social factors in ASPD comes from cross-cultural research, with highly persuasive data from East Asia. Samples from urban and rural areas of Taiwan (Compton et al. 1991; Hwu et al. 1989) demonstrated an unusually low prevalence of ASPD: less than 0.2%. These rates also apply to mainland China (Cheung 1991) and Japan (Sato and Takeichi 1993) but not to South Korea (Lee et al. 1987).

The East Asian cultures with a low prevalence of ASPD have cultural and family structures that are strongly protective against antisocial behavior. They maintain high levels of cohesion through traditional family and social structures. These families are a veritable mirror image of the risk factors for psychopathy: fathers are strong and authoritative, expectations of children are high, and family loyalty is prized. The Robins (1966) study found a particularly low rate of ASPD in Jewish subjects, which was attributed to their strong family structures. It is also possible that the repressive style seen in some traditional families may have a different association: with personality disorders in the C cluster (Paris 1998b).

Clinical Implications

The pathways to ASPD help us to understand the problematic course and treatment of this disorder. Patients with ASPD are unusually impulsive (and/or readily behaviorally activated), traits that modulate only slowly over time. These characteristics are exaggerated by feedback loops with the environment. Because social and/or family dysfunction amplify traits, these patterns are difficult to change without making major modifications to the social milieu. Moreover, patients with ASPD often seek out environments (such as criminal gangs) that reinforce their deviance.

Of all the personality disorders, the antisocial category offers the most pessimistic prospects for treatment. Attempts to treat patients with ASPD have generally involved individual and group therapies or "therapeutic communities" (Lykken 1995). However, there is no evidence that any of these methods produces any lasting effects. (See Chapter 8 for a more detailed discussion.)

Borderline Personality Disorder

BPD has become a major focus of clinical attention in recent decades. This disorder may have been given different diagnoses in the past, but indirect evidence, based on documented increases in characteristic symptoms such as repetitive parasuicide, suggests that the prevalence of BPD in the community is increasing (Millon 1993; Paris 1996). The precise estimate of prevalence varies widely from study to study, owing to variations in samples and methods. A Norwegian survey found a rate of 4% (Bodlund et al. 1993), whereas Lenzenweger et al. (1997) were unable to find any cases in a sample of American college students. Using data from the ECA study to reconstruct the borderline diagnosis, Swartz et al. (1990) estimated a prevalence of 1.8%. The median prevalence across all studies is 1.1% (Mattia and Zimmerman 2001), but the most recent studies suggest that the true rate might be even less. Torgersen et al. (2001) found a rate of 0.7% in their study in Oslo, Norway. Although Samuels et al. (2002) obtained a rate of 1.2%, when the rate was weighted to reflect differences between the sample and the population, it went down to 0.5%. The prevalence of BPD may also vary from one setting to another, depending on levels of social change and disruption, consistent with the social sensitivity of impulsive disorders discussed in Chapter 1.

Biological Factors

Siever and Davis (1991) hypothesized that the personality dimensions underlying BPD are impulsivity and affective instability. Many patients with BPD also show a third dimension of pathology: cognitive impairment associated with micropsychotic phenomena (Zanarini et al. 1990). All three dimensions are established to be heritable (Jang et al. 1996).

Impulsivity is the most researched of these traits. It has a robust relationship to decreased central serotonin activity (Mann 1998). Similar findings have emerged using several different methods: peripheral measures of serotonin levels in platelets (Kavoussi and Coccaro 1998), serotonin metabolites in cerebrospinal fluid (Mann 1998), challenge tests in which agonists stimulate brain serotonin (Gurvits et al. 2000), and positron emission tomography studies with serotonin agonists (Leyton et al. 2001). Specific serotonin reuptake inhibitors have some effect (albeit not a dramatic one) in reducing impulsive symptoms in patients with BPD (Coccaro and Kavoussi 1997). Finally, as in ASPD, patients with BPD have neuropsychological deficits in executive function, which is located in the prefrontal cortex (O'Leary 2000).

Much less is known about the nature of affective instability in BPD (and even less about cognitive symptoms). Patients with BPD respond with strong emotion to life events and take more time to come back to a baseline state. They also have unusually high levels of neuroticism (Costa and Widiger 1994), although this trait is also high in Cluster C personality disorders (Brieger et al. 2000; Zweig-Frank and Paris 1995). Linehan et al. (1993) emphasized an intrinsically high level of emotional lability that treatment methods can target and modify. Siever and Davis (1991) hypothesized that affective lability is modulated by neurochemical pathways involving noradrenergic and cholinergic systems.

Psychological Factors

Most (but not all) patients with BPD describe serious adversities during childhood (Paris 1994). The most common are family dysfunction, serious parental pathology (such as antisocial personality and substance abuse), childhood abuse, and neglect (Zanarini et al. 1990).

Although retrospective reports of childhood experiences can be accurate (Brewin 1996), they are colored by recall bias (Maughan and Rutter 1997; Schacter 1996). An interesting example of how events at one stage of life can be remembered very differently at another stage emerged in a recent study by Offer et al. (2000). A cohort of asymptomatic adolescents, originally interviewed in the 1960s (described in Chapter 1), were followed into middle age. There was no relationship between how the subjects remembered their teenage years (particularly family relationships) and how they reported their circumstances at the time. We cannot take childhood histories in adult patients at face value.

Despite these difficulties, strong converging data from several sources support the relationship between childhood adversity and borderline personality. In a sample of untreated volunteers with BPD (Salzman et al. 1993), as well in a sample of 50-year-old former patients with BPD from our follow-up study (Zweig-Frank and Paris 2002), subjects reported high rates of childhood trauma. Tellingly, abuse and neglect are also associated with a higher rate of personality disorder symptoms in community samples (J.J. Johnson et al. 1999). As described in Chapter 3, abuse and neglect have been *directly* documented in the childhoods of children with borderline pathology. Finally, the risk factors for BPD closely parallel those established in prospective research on ASPD (Robins 1966): parental sociopathy, family dysfunction, and inconsistent discipline.

Thus, there can be little question that trauma and neglect during childhood are *risk factors* for borderline pathology. However, this does not prove that childhood adversity is the primary *cause* of the disorder.

First, no specificity exists between risk factors and sequelae. The psychological risk factors associated with BPD (child abuse, neglect, dysfunctional families, and parental psychopathology) are neither consistent nor universal. In our own large-scale study of women and men with BPD (Paris et al. 1994a, 1994b), only about one-third of the subjects described severe childhood trauma. This portion of the sample had experienced multiple adversities in the course of development, with accordingly greater long-term risk (Rutter 1989). For this group, it was safe to assume that childhood trauma had a strong influence on adult functioning. However, another third of our subjects reported only a moderate degree of early adversity. Many reported less specific problems such as unempathic parents and/or isolated incidents of sexual or physical abuse. Finally, about one-third of our subjects had *no* significant history of childhood adversity. We interpreted these findings in the light of the stress–diathesis model presented in Chapter 1. Some subjects had experienced high levels of adversity that interacted with predispositions to cause serious psychopathology. Others had experienced low levels of adversity but were sufficiently vulnerable to be "tipped over" by much lower levels of stress.

The second issue is that childhood adversity, by itself, does not predictably lead to personality disorders. As discussed in Chapter 3, experiences of abuse and neglect are found in asymptomatic community populations. Community studies often show high levels of resilience in children with traumatic childhoods (Paris 2000c; Rutter and Rutter 1993).

Third, trauma and neglect are reported by a wide variety of patients with very different symptoms. Most likely, childhood adversities are risk factors for many types of personality disorders. In our own studies, all reported adversities in BPD overlapped with the comparison group (patients with other Axis II diagnoses, mainly in the C cluster). Histories of childhood trauma are also common in depression and other Axis I disorders (Bifulco et al. 1991). This nonlinear relationship between childhood experiences and adult psychopathology can be explained through interactions with temperament. Personality disorders would develop only in vulnerable individuals, and specific disorders would be associated with specific traits. Thus, BPD would require the prior presence of impulsivity and affective instability. Abuse and neglect would make temperamentally impulsive children even more impulsive and could also exaggerate affective lability.

Social Factors

Impulsivity and affective instability are "socially sensitive" traits. Therefore, the prevalence of BPD should show strong cohort effects as well as cross-cultural differences (Paris 1996). Although ASPD was the only personality disorder studied in the ECA study and NCS, the prevalence of BPD will be directly assessed in the forthcoming NCS Replication and International Comorbidity Study. This research will provide us with measurements of regional and cross-national differences.

At present, a good deal of indirect evidence points to an association between social stressors and BPD. Increases in prevalence for this disorder over recent decades are suggested by increases in rates of youth suicide and parasuicide (Paris 1996), especially given that one-third of suicidal youth can be found to have BPD (Lesage et al. 1994).

The social factors affecting the prevalence of BPD may be similar to those previously described for ASPD. Disorders characterized by impulsivity and affective instability should tend to increase when there is a higher rate of family breakdown, when there is a loss of social cohesion, and when social roles are less readily available (Paris 1996). However, such stressors would have their strongest effects on those who are temperamentally vulnerable.

Clinical Implications

Feedback loops between temperament and experience shape the development of BPD and also contribute to its chronicity. Patients with BPD fall into vicious circles that interfere with their ability to work and to love, and these feedback loops further feed impulsivity and instability. Moreover, the partners of these patients may also have Cluster B personality disorders (Paris and Braverman 1995).

We see these interactions when we treat patients with BPD. They are difficult to engage because of impulsivity and, once in treatment, difficult to soothe because of affective lability. It is therefore not surprising that many therapists describe frustrating experiences treating these patients. Sometimes we do not recognize the nature of borderline pathology, and the ensuing turmoil that engulfs therapy comes as a surprise. Sometimes we are misled by an initial idealization and connection with the patient's neediness (a "rescue fantasy") and are dispirited by the devaluation and splitting that come later.

Naturalistic studies of the treatment of BPD (Buckley et al. 1981; Skodol et al. 1983; Waldinger and Gunderson 1984) have observed high dropout rates, approaching two-thirds of all patients who enter treatment. One reason may be that unstructured therapies are not tailored to the special needs of patients with BPD. As Chapter 8 shows, patients with BPD tend to do better in highly structured environments, such as day treatment programs (Bateman and Fonagy 2001; Piper et al. 1996), or highly structured outpatient therapy (Linehan 1993, 1999).

Some of the difficulty that clinicians have with patients who have BPD derives from a failure to take the chronicity of the disorder into account. Over the years, some therapists have claimed, without much evidence, that they have a definitive way of treating patients who have BPD. In my view, clinicians do better by setting their sights lower, avoiding unreasonable expectations for full recovery. (This issue is discussed further in Chapter 8.)

The comorbidity associated with BPD adds another confusing set of problems to management. Mood symptoms in BPD tend to be chronic, often beginning with early onset dysthymia (Pepper et al. 1995), and depression does not respond predictably to pharmacotherapy (Gunderson and Phillips 1991). Patients with Cluster B personality disorders often abuse drugs (Robins 1966; Zanarini 2000), and patients with substance abuse often have Axis II comorbidity (Nace and Davis 1993). Although patients with BPD can behave (e.g., cutting themselves) in an addictive, repetitive way yet still manage to function in work or school, the same cannot be said about patients with substance abuse. Those who stop are more likely to recover from personality disturbance, whereas those who cannot will fall down the social scale, not infrequently dying young. Chapter 5 documents the effects of substance abuse on the outcome of BPD.

Narcissistic Personality Disorder

Patients with narcissistic personality disorder (NPD) are frequently seen in psychiatric practices. Although the nature of narcissistic pathology is not well understood, a similar model to those described above for ASPD and BPD can be applied to NPD.

Biological Factors

Little is known about the biological factors in NPD, but like any other personality disorder, it should have roots in temperament. Narcissism as a trait has a heritable component (Jang et al. 1998), and in the Oslo twin sample (Torgersen et al. 2000), as much as 77% of the variance in NPD was attributable to genetic factors. We do not know *what* is being inherited, but temperamental characteristics could influence personality traits such as needs for approval and attention.

Psychological Factors

Kohut (1970) believed that pathological narcissism arises from consistent defects in parental empathy. He hypothesized that children respond to such failures by becoming defensively grandiose and/or withdrawn. This model ("self psychology") has been influential, largely because it encouraged therapists to treat patients with warmth and empathy. However, Kohut's ideas have never been tested empirically. If everyone who was consistently misunderstood by their parents reacted in the same way, we would *all* be narcissistic. (Kohut might even have agreed with this conclusion.)

Narcissistic personality traits can be identified in childhood (Guilé 2000). These children may require unusual levels of sensitivity, as well as careful limit setting, from their parents. Otherwise, feedback loops tend to develop that will amplify these traits to pathological proportions. When a child with strong narcissistic needs demands understanding that is not available and/or misbehaves in ways that are not contained, the trait will be exaggerated. Finally, people are more likely to be self-regarding and grandiose when they have some unusual or desirable characteristics, such as intelligence or beauty, but people with narcissistic traits always seem to find *something* about themselves that is special.

Social Factors

Although we have no good community studies of cohort effects on prevalence, many clinicians describe seeing more patients with NPD. This could simply be a matter of perception, reflecting the way therapists formulate their cases. However, it is also possible that NPD may actually be becoming more common. Social networks are much less cohesive in modern society. The absence of these structures fails to channel narcissistic traits into fruitful ambition. Individuals with these characteristics might therefore be more likely to develop personality disorders. Alternatively, it may be that narcissism has not changed but its consequences have. In traditional society, family and community buffer the effects of personal selfishness. In modern society, interpersonal relationships are less stable, and those who fail to invest in them are more likely to become socially isolated.

Clinical Implications

We have little formal data on the therapy for NPD (see Chapter 8), but clinical experience suggests that these patients provide a quintessential example of why personality disorders can be difficult to treat. Narcissistic traits interfere directly with the process of psychotherapy. Grandiosity leads them to resist acknowledging personal responsibility for problems. Arrogance interferes with the formation of a therapeutic alliance. Entitlement leads to unreasonable demands on therapists. Thus, patients with NPD have a reputation for intransigence. The chances of success may be better when patients are clinically depressed or, as Kernberg (1976) once suggested, when they reach middle age.

Avoidant Personality Disorder

Patients with Cluster C personality disorders are common in both clinical and community populations (Mattia and Zimmerman 2001). The category with the most empirical data is avoidant personality disorder (APD).

Biological Factors

A large body of research shows that anxious traits are heritable (see review in Paris 1998a). If APD is a pathological exaggeration of such traits, it should also show genetic influence. The twin study by Torgersen et al. (2000) shows that this is indeed the case, with 28% of the variance being accounted for by heritable factors.

Kagan (1994) described children with high levels of *behavioral inhibition*— that is, unusual fearfulness from very early in childhood. Follow-up study of these cohorts has shown continued anxiety in adolescence, associated with early onset biological markers for trait anxiety, including rapid heart rate and increased autonomic sensitivity. As discussed in Chapter 2, these symptoms could be precursors of APD.

Psychological Factors

Patients with APD may describe overprotective parenting during childhood (Head et al. 1991). Although parents are unlikely to be the main cause of the disorder, overprotection probably plays a role in amplifying temperamental vulnerability. Shy children elicit these responses, whereas impulsive children would not allow themselves to be dealt with in this way. When parents are overprotective, children lose the opportunity to be exposed to what they fear and to tolerate and master social anxiety. If this feedback loop is not broken, social development may be crippled.

Social Factors

In a traditional social setting, anxious traits need not lead to serious problems, because family and community members are available to "cover" for unusually shy individuals. However, it is more difficult for shy children to cope in modern society, with its low cohesion and less accessible social roles (Paris 1998a). As a result, anxious traits may become socially disabling and lead to diagnosable disorders.

Clinical Implications

We know little about the treatment of APD, other than a few trials of social skills training for selected patients (see Chapter 8). The main problem in the management of APD is that the disorder is self-reinforcing. Failure to master social skills can lead to increasing isolation, producing long-term distress and chronicity.

   I also suspect that patients with APD avoid the mental health system. In my experience in a community consultation clinic, I see surprisingly few patients with APD coming for treatment. Yet Torgersen et al. (2001) found a high community prevalence (5%) in their Oslo sample. Some of these patients could be receiving behavioral or cognitive-behavioral therapy for an overlapping diagnosis on Axis I of generalized social phobia. Others may simply be avoiding treatment entirely.

Other Personality Disorders

Cluster A

In Chapter 2, I described evidence for a common predisposition to schizophrenia and to the personality disorders in the schizophrenic spectrum. I also presented hypotheses, based on a stress–diathesis model, as to why some patients develop psychosis whereas others do not.

Of the three disorders in the A cluster, the largest body of research is about schizotypal personality disorder. However, most published articles have focused on biological factors shared between this Axis II disorder and schizophrenia. Little has been written about what these patients are like in clinical settings. This situation is about to change, because the National Institute of Mental Health (NIMH) Collaborative Study of Personality Disorders is following a cohort of schizotypal patients who are being compared to groups with BPD, APD, and obsessive-compulsive personality disorder (OCPD). The greatest functional impairment was observed in patients with borderline and schizotypal pathology (Skodol et al. 2002), and these were also the patients who used the most treatment resources (Bender et al. 2001). However, there may be many patients with schizotypal pathology who are not connected with the mental health system, and Torgersen et al. (2001) found nearly as many patients with schizotypal pathology as with BPD in his Oslo sample. In my experience, patients with schizotypal traits who do present to the mental health system can suffer, in much the same way as those with schizophrenia, from loneliness and marginalization. Chapter 8 discusses how these problems can be addressed in treatment.

Cluster B

Only one category in this group has not been discussed above: histrionic personality disorder (HPD). There are very few articles in the literature with empirical data specifically related to HPD. In Chapter 2 I reviewed data on its epidemiology and heritability and suggested how this disorder might be understood in a stress–diathesis model. Unfortunately, we know little about the course or the treatment of HPD. Chapter 5 presents some clinical speculations about its outcome.

Cluster C

Dependent personality disorder has little empirical literature. In the Oslo survey (Torgersen et al. 2001), its prevalence was 1.5%; Torgersen et al. (2000) observed heritability to be 0.57. As defined by DSM-IV-TR (American Psychiatric Association 2000), the disorder seems to be somewhat more common in women (Bornstein 1997; Loranger 1996). In my opinion, the construct is somewhat shaky, in that dependent personality disorder is defined almost exclusively in terms of one exaggerated trait and, as suggested in Chapter 2, the distinction between the avoidant and dependent categories is unclear.

We can expect to know more about OCPD in the future; this category is one of the four undergoing follow-up evaluation by the NIMH Collaborative Study of Personality Disorders. In the Oslo survey by Torgersen et al. (2001), its prevalence was 2%; in the twin study by Torgersen et al. (2000), the heritability was 0.78. As discussed in Chapter 2, OCPD might be understood in a stress–diathesis model, with compulsivity as a heritable trait that can be amplified to pathological proportions under stressful life circumstances.

Results from the NIMH Collaborative Study indicate thus far that patients with OCPD are less impaired than those in the borderline or schizotypal categories (Skodol et al. 2002). Although they use mental health services less often than those with more severe disorders, they were noted to be high consumers of psychotherapy (Bender et al. 2001). (One wonders if this is because those with compulsive personalities have difficulty accepting less-than-perfect results, even in therapy.)

Traits, Course, and Outcome

The model of personality disorders presented in this chapter can account for their course and outcome. Ultimately, the chronicity of disorders reflects the stability of underlying traits. Research has consistently shown that as people grow older, their personality gradually becomes more fixed. Moreover, because personality determines how we interact with our environment, existing traits are consistently reinforced, for good or for ill, through stable feedback loops.

The most extensive study of the relationship between personality and aging was conducted by Costa and McCrae (1988) at Johns Hopkins University. In childhood and adolescence, significant personality change is possible. Impulsive children can "straighten out," and shy children can overcome social anxiety. After age 18, however, personality becomes much more constant, and after age 30, it hardly changes.

The course of time, as well as psychotherapy, may soften or modify traits but rarely produces basic change. Because trait profiles are stable, they tend to predict future life course. In a 45-year follow-up study of college men, Soldz and Vaillant (1999) found that high levels of neuroticism in youth were associated with increased difficulties later in life, whereas high levels of conscientiousness predicted success.

Most people come to accept that as adults, they must work their way around whatever traits they have. However, patients with personality disorders face a dilemma. Their coping strategies are narrow and fixed, and they tend to repeat the same mistakes in different forms, over and over again. This raises the question as to how therapists can help patients with personality disorders. We know that patients with Axis II diagnoses are formidable consumers of mental health services (Bender et al. 2001), yet our methods for treating them are at an early stage of development. We do not, at this point, have drugs that can change personality. Therapy focusing on the impact of childhood experiences does not yield predictable results, because understanding the past will not necessarily break well-established feedback loops continuing into the present. We can note the impact of social circumstances on personality pathology, but this does not necessarily point to a way out for individuals. Instead, we need to consider ways to help patients use their traits in more effective ways. This is discussed in Chapter 10.

5

Long-Term Outcome of Personality Disorders

Antisocial Personality Disorder

Patients with antisocial personality disorder (ASPD) have a grim future. The course of ASPD is chronic, almost malignant, and we would expect its long-term outcome to be equally poor. However, there have been only a few formal follow-up studies of patients with ASPD. The reason is the difficulty in obtaining compliance from this population for research. These are people who can turn up when they are in trouble and then disappear for a long time.

The first formal assessment of the outcome of ASPD was conducted by Robins (1966), whose large-scale study included a follow-up component. Within the relatively brief time frame of 5 years, Robins followed 82 subjects, reporting that in 12% the disorder had remitted, 27% had experienced improvement, and 61% had experienced no improvement. The study also found a suicide rate of 5%, a finding that suggests that patients with ASPD are not as immune from depression as clinicians have thought.

A few years later, Maddocks (1970) reported on a British follow-up study of patients with ASPD. Of 59 men drawn from an outpatient setting, fewer than 20% had experienced improvement over a 5-year period. However, this study had some obvious limitations: The ratings were global and the time frame was short.

Another strand of evidence comes from forensic settings. Although not all patients with ASPD become involved in the criminal justice system, there is a high rate of ASPD in prison populations (Robins and Regier 1991). Because it is well established that criminal convictions decline with time (Arboleda-Flores 1991), the impulsivity associated with ASPD may burn out.

This conjecture has been confirmed by one comprehensive study of the long-term outcome of ASPD. This landmark research was carried out by a team led by Don Black, a psychiatrist at the University of Iowa. Black et al. (1995) reported on 71 men with a diagnosis of ASPD documented during admission to a psychiatric hospital in Iowa City between 1945 and 1970. The cohort was followed for periods ranging from 16 to 45 years. Black and colleagues acknowledged that their group was not precisely representative of the population with ASPD, most of whom have never been admitted to psychiatric hospitals. However, the advantage of using this cohort lay in the collection of detailed records, allowing the team to be certain that all subjects met diagnostic criteria for ASPD at baseline.

Not surprisingly, tracing these men presented a major challenge. Many had left the state, were not in contact with their relatives, or were living in marginal circumstances. One of the more interesting findings was that 17 of 71 had died prematurely (Black et al. 1996). This high mortality rate, almost one-quarter of those traced, resembles that of substance abusers (Vaillant 1995).

Nor were the men in this cohort easy to interview. Patients with ASPD are well known for lying. In this study, nearly 30% of the sample denied all past difficulties, even criminal offenses that had been documented in great detail. Some of the subjects were located in prison. A few were inebriated at the time of the interview. One even physically threatened the research assistant. Finally, one man, like the condemned criminal in the film *Dead Man Walking*, made sexually suggestive remarks to his female interviewer.

In spite of all these difficulties, the team was able to trace all but 3 of the 71 men. Of the 68 who were found, only 36 agreed to be contacted, and only 26 of these agreed to a formal interview. Information from key informants allowed researchers to make partial assessments of 9 more subjects.

Of this total of 45 subjects, 19 were rated as having unimproved pathology, 14 as having improved but not remitted pathology, and 12 as having experienced full remission. Among the 21 men formally interviewed (using the Diagnostic Interview Schedule), only in 2 did pathology still merit a current diagnosis of ASPD. This finding was largely due to a reduction in impulsivity. Even among those who no longer met formal criteria, many continued to have severe problems in close interpersonal relationships. Most of these individuals would probably still have met general criteria for a personality disorder, as described in DSM-IV-TR (American Psychiatric Association 2000). In categorical terms, one might say they had graduated from the specific category of ASPD to a diagnosis of personality disorder not otherwise specified.

All subjects in this cohort had been married at some point, with 61% married at the time of follow-up evaluation, and with 39% having had more than one wife. Notably, as many as 91% of the cohort had produced children. As Stone (1990) suggested, the successfully predatory behavior of men with ASPD toward women may have the effect of keeping these traits in the gene pool. On the other hand, few of these men actually raised their children. Moreover, about one-third of the offspring were reported to have psychiatric disturbances. Finally, the cohort demonstrated serious deficits in their work histories. About one-quarter were unemployed when interviewed, and almost one-half had been irregularly employed. Not surprisingly, substance abuse was an important predictor of outcome. There was a statistically significant relationship between current alcoholism and remission: Of the 12 individuals who were presently alcoholic, none had experienced remission of their disorder.

The study by Black's team, which overcame almost insuperable obstacles to follow-up research, will likely be one of a kind for some time to come. Its most provocative finding was that recovery from an impulsive personality disorder does not imply full psychological remission. Instead, although patients with ASPD are less likely to commit crimes or carry out impulsive acts as they grow older, they continue to be very difficult people. Over the years, they remain poor spouses, inadequate parents, and unsteady workers.

Borderline Personality Disorder

Samples and Settings

Borderline personality disorder (BPD) is famously chronic. In a memorable phrase, Schmideberg (1959) described its course as "stably unstable." These clinical impressions have been confirmed by research. Moreover, instability tends to continue in spite of intensive efforts at treatment. For many of the researchers who have followed these patients, most of whom are committed psychotherapists, the long-term outcome for BPD has been sobering. (This may be one reason why some research has gone unpublished.)

The first formal follow-up studies of patients with BPD were conducted in the 1970s. Three research groups, at Michael Reese Hospital in Chicago (Werble 1970), at the National Institute of Mental Health (NIMH; Carpenter et al. 1977), and at McLean Hospital outside Boston (Pope et al. 1983), examined cohorts 5 years after initial presentation. In each case, the essential findings were that patients with BPD had changed very little within 5 years, but this is too brief a period to determine the outcome of a chronic disorder.

As described in the Introduction, a series of multiple (and serendipitous) 15-year follow-up studies of patients with BPD were carried out in the

1980s. The results of these studies are summarized and compared in Table 5–1.

The Chestnut Lodge study (McGlashan 1986a) described a cohort treated at a famous (and expensive) private hospital near Washington, D.C. This was the real-life setting for Joanne Greenberg's autobiographical novel, *I Never Promised You a Rose Garden*, later turned into a successful film. Its most famous therapist had been the redoubtable Frieda Fromm-Reichmann, who was Greenberg's therapist. Although Greenberg was considered at the time to have schizophrenia, her symptoms (characterized by an intense fantasy of living on another planet) met criteria for BPD. Unlike the patients with schizophrenia in the Chestnut Lodge sample, Greenberg made a full and early recovery from her illness; today she is a highly functional professional writer.

Patients at "the Lodge" were often admitted for several years to receive intensive psychotherapy in a residential setting. In the period after World War II, this was considered an avant-garde method. This practice underwent a major modification in the 1980s, after the Osheroff case (Klerman 1990), in which a physician sued the Lodge after having been treated there for 6 months with psychotherapy only, and then recovering dramatically after receiving medication at another hospital.

Stone (1990) followed a similar but larger cohort of patients treated at the New York State Psychiatric Institute. This large psychiatric hospital associated with Columbia University has focused on the treatment of psychosis, but in the 1950s and 1960s it maintained a ward that functioned as a residential treatment center offering intensive psychotherapy for troubled young people. Unlike Chestnut Lodge, the state paid for long-term inpatient treatment, so that the institute's long-term ward was open to middle-class patients. In practice, however, the cohort was largely upper class, selected either from private therapy practices or from VIP referrals.

A third cohort was drawn from patients admitted to Austen Riggs Hospital (Plakun et al. 1985). This famous private hospital in the Berkshires, which once had Erik Erikson on staff, resembles Chestnut Lodge, both in its history and in its orientation.

The fourth study was based on a general hospital cohort in Montreal (Paris et al. 1987). This sample, drawn from an urban hospital, stood in contrast to the privileged and highly educated groups in the other studies. (By the 1960s, in Canada, inpatient treatment was already paid for by the government.) Thus, half of our cohort had never finished high school, and most came from the middle and lower end of the social spectrum. This profile closely resembles that of patients with BPD seen in most clinics, as well as the social class distribution found in epidemiological studies of BPD (Swartz et al. 1990). Another contrast to the other studies, in which almost

TABLE 5–1. Long-term studies of the outcome of borderline personality disorder

Site	Chestnut Lodge (private)	Columbia (state)	Austen Riggs (private)	Montreal (private)
Years of follow-up monitoring	15	15	15	15 and 27
Percent cohort located	86	91	27	32 and 26
Number assessed	81	206	54	100 and 64
Mean age	47	37	40	39 and 51
Percent male vs. female	46 vs. 54	30 vs. 70	27 vs. 73	16 vs. 84 and 17 vs. 83
Socioeconomic status	High	High	High	Wide range
Percent ever married	70	Women, 52%; men, 29%	?	67
Percent with children	48	Women, 25%; men, 15%	?	59
Mean Global Assessment of Functioning score	64	67	67	63 and 63
Percent still having borderline personality disorder	?	?	?	25 and 8
Percent dead by means other than suicide	13	13	?	13 and 18
Percent dead by suicide	3	9	?	9 and 10
Mean age (years) at suicide	?	30	?	30 and 37
Outcome predictors	IQ (+), length previous admissions (−), affective instability (−)	IQ (+), child abuse (−)	Self-harm (+), anger (+)	Dysthymia (−), problems with mother (−)
Suicide predictors	?	Substance abuse (+), major depression (+)	?	Previous attempts (+), education (+)

Note. + = positive correlation; − = negative correlation; ? = not reported.

all patients were in long-term outpatient psychotherapy, was that the treatment histories in our group were extremely variable. Only a minority had received intensive therapy, and most had been seen either briefly or intermittently by a psychotherapist.

A fifth group, at Mount Sinai Hospital in Toronto, conducted a 10-year follow-up study of patients with BPD (Silver and Cardish 1991). Their ward, also located in a general hospital, functioned very much like the one at Columbia—that is, as a residential setting where patients could live for years while receiving intensive psychotherapy. Sadly, the results of the Toronto follow-up study were never published. However, I do refer to the major findings of this study, which were presented at a meeting of the American Psychiatric Association, later in the chapter.

Methodologies

Strictly speaking, none of the five follow-up studies of BPD was truly prospective. Instead, baseline diagnoses were established retrospectively from chart review data, applying current diagnostic criteria. However, because the information in the charts was extensive (as it tended to be in those days), one can feel some degree of confidence that these baseline diagnoses were correct.

Subjects in all the groups were monitored into early middle age (around age 40 years). The sample sizes in the main studies were sufficient to carry out multiple statistical analyses: 81 for McGlashan (1986a), 193 for Stone (1990), 63 for Plakun et al. (1985), and 100 in our group (Paris et al. 1987). In all of these studies, about 80% of the subjects were female.

The percentage of located subjects varied greatly. McGlashan and Stone had the highest rates (over 80%). Their success in finding patients was an enormous advantage because attrition can play havoc with the validity of results in follow-up research. In contrast, the other studies did much less well. For example, Plakun's group succeeded in locating less than one-third of its original cohort. Our own group succeeded in locating only one-half of the patients who had been identified by chart review, and in the end, we interviewed only about one-third of that total. Many of the subjects we were searching for had spent only a short time in hospital. Thus, our cohort did not have the level of institutional attachment that aided studies based on residential treatment. According to McGlashan, former patients would say to his interviewers, "Oh, you're from the Lodge—I was wondering when you would finally call!"

When researchers conducting follow-up studies cannot find subjects, they may carry out bias testing comparing located and nonlocated individuals. The researchers who did this (McGlashan, Plakun et al., Paris et al.) found few or no differences from baseline data. However, one can never be sure whether the missing subjects might not have differed in important ways on outcome measures.

Three studies (McGlashan, Stone, Paris et al.) assessed outcome largely through telephone interviews. Although there could be qualitative losses using this method, McGlashan took the trouble to compare data obtained from face-to-face interviews with those from phone interviews and found no differences. In Stone's study, not everyone was interviewed, and in some cases functioning was assessed from reports by key informants. (As we saw in the study by Black et al. [1995] of ASPD, ex-patients are not always interested in talking to researchers.) Finally, the study by Plakun et al. limited its assessment to mailed questionnaires.

Thus, each study had its own limitations. In one way or another, each suffered from a bias in the sample or a problem in measurement. Yet these problems may have canceled each other out. Thus, although McGlashan's study was the soundest methodologically, its subjects differed from the patients with BPD whom most clinicians see. In contrast, although our Montreal study failed to locate the majority of potential subjects, its sample was more representative of the population with BPD. In the end, all studies of the outcome of patients with BPD reported almost *identical* results. This concordance among different studies was striking and remarkable. We can therefore be reasonably confident about the conclusions.

Results

All studies measured global outcome at follow-up evaluation, using variants of the same measure: the Health-Sickness Rating Scale (HSRS; Luborsky 1963), the Global Adaptation Scale (GAS; Endicott et al. 1976), which was the basis for the Axis V scale published in the various editions of DSM (also called the Global Assessment of Functioning (GAF) scale). All studies also assessed specific outcomes: work, relationships, symptomatology, and further hospitalization. Our report was the only one to specifically examine whether patients still met formal criteria for BPD. For this purpose, we used a semistructured interview measure developed at McLean Hospital, the Diagnostic Interview for Borderlines (DIB-R; Zanarini et al. 1989).

Global outcome scores were nearly identical in all studies, with means falling in the mid-60s. (An HSRS or GAF score in this range reflects mild difficulties and can be considered as lying within the broad range of normality.) Rehospitalization was uncommon after the first few years in all the cohorts. By the time of follow-up evaluation, most patients were working and had a reasonable social life. Our study also found that only 25% of the original sample still met diagnostic criteria for BPD. All the subscales of the DIB-R—dysphoria, impulsivity, disturbed relationships, and micropsychotic phenomena—showed improvement over time.

Thus far, the results seem quite encouraging—surprisingly so, given the depth of pathology these patients had at baseline. However, the downside to the story was the high rate of completed suicide. Both Stone's study and our own reported rates close to 9%. McGlashan's cohort had a much lower rate, only 3%. Does this indicate that treatment at Chestnut Lodge was uniquely effective, more so than at other hospitals? McGlashan stated that he would like to believe so but considers another explanation more likely. Patients admitted to Chestnut Lodge, unlike those seen at Columbia or Montreal, were sifted from those for whom treatment in general hospitals failed, and were somewhat older. Thus, some of the patients most at risk might have already died by suicide.

Other studies have confirmed the high frequency of suicide in patients with BPD. In Oslo, Norway, 291 patients with BPD were identified from a psychiatric clinic at the university. When their names were searched for in the National Death Cause Registry, it was found that 23 (14 men and 9 women) had committed suicide, giving a rate of 8% (Kjelsberg et al. 1991). Another study of residential treatment in Norway (Aarkrog 1993; presented at a conference but unfortunately unpublished) reported a 10% suicide rate. Finally, the unpublished Toronto study by Silver and Cardish found that 7 of 70 (10%) had died by suicide by the 10-year follow-up point.

In summary, we can conclude with some degree of confidence that about 1 in 10 patients with BPD will eventually go on to complete suicide. This rate is not very different from that found in patients with schizophrenia (Wilkinson 1982) and in those with major mood disorders (Guze and Robins 1970).

All of the studies that examined suicide found a disproportionate number of males (about half) among the completers, in spite of the fact that at least three-quarters of patients with BPD are female. This should not be surprising, given the well-known preponderance of males among those who complete suicide.

Under what conditions do patients with BPD end their lives? At the 15-year follow-up point, most of the suicide completions in our study, as well as in Stone's, had occurred within the first 5 years of follow-up study, with a mean age at death of about 30 years. However, contrary to common fears of clinicians, suicides tended not to occur either while patients were in active therapy or following a stormy visit to the emergency department. Instead, patients committed suicide after many years of unsuccessful therapy, often when they were no longer in treatment.

The other side of this story is good news: Most patients with BPD, even those who had been chronically suicidal for years, remained alive. Given the global outcome findings, it seems that patients who have BPD and who do not kill themselves can be expected to experience improved functioning over time.

Nonetheless, the survivors may be better described as functionally improved than as "recovered." When we go beyond quantitative data and consider results from a qualitative point of view, the outcome of BPD looks less rosy. Our clinical impression, which agrees with those of both McGlashan and Silver and Cardish, is that many former patients with BPD remain fragile and continue to demonstrate some degree of impairment. Even when levels of global functioning are satisfactory, their lives can remain restricted and unfulfilled. (This will more apparent later, when I discuss our 27-year follow-up findings.)

One example of long-term sequelae in BPD is family life. Stone found that only 52% of the females with BPD had married, whereas only 25% had ever had children. Among the males, as few as 29% had married, and only 15% had had children. (This contrasts with the relative fecundity of men with ASPD in the sample of Black et al.) Among those who did marry, there was no evidence of an unusually high divorce rate (only one-third by age 40 years, not excessive compared with national averages). However, of those whose marriages broke down, only 10% eventually remarried (less than national averages). As is described below, the results for our own sample were similar, with less than half marrying, and fewer bearing children. McGlashan's (1986a) cohort had a higher rate of marriage (70%), possibly reflecting a less severely ill cohort.

In Chapter 7 I provide examples of how stable intimacy can be protective for patients with BPD. I also describe how being responsible for a child can blunt the sharp edge of impulsivity. Patients with BPD who become mothers may lose their diagnosis but retain enough symptoms to meet criteria for personality disorder not otherwise specified.

Yet marriage and children are not for everyone. Bardenstein and McGlashan (1989) expressed concern about the value of intimate relationships in patients with BPD, remarking that "marriage for borderline women more often than not provided an arena for the enactment of psychopathology" (p. 79). Examining the Chestnut Lodge sample, they found that women with BPD actually had a somewhat poorer long-term outcome than men did, a gender difference that could be attributed to marital disturbances. Moreover, women with BPD became increasingly symptomatic in their 40s if their marriages broke down, sometimes developing alcoholism. These findings, pointing to continued fragility in late middle age, with symptoms presenting a kind of "U curve" over time, led McGlashan (personal communication, 1991) to recommend a longer follow-up period for BPD.

Predictors of Outcome

Because every patient is unique, predicting outcome for an individual can be perilous. Nonetheless, researchers must attempt to determine, at least at the group level, what influences risk for a poor global outcome or for suicide. Among possible predictive factors might be functional level before treatment, the presence of particular symptom patterns, education, or developmental experiences.

McGlashan (1985) reported that his two strongest predictors of positive outcome were higher intelligence and shorter length of previous hospitalization. However, neither of these factors accounted for a large percentage of the outcome variance. Nor were they highly specific, because these variables are predictive of the outcome of almost any psychiatric disorder. This is a specific example of a general problem: Predictors can be statistically significant yet may not be clinically useful.

Do patients with one type of symptom do better than patients with a different pattern? The only clinical predictor in McGlashan's (1985) study that was specific to BPD was affective instability, a symptom that predicted a negative outcome. Our group (Paris et al. 1988) reported a similar finding, although mood symptoms did not account for much of the outcome variance. Plakun et al. (1985) had reported the paradoxical observation that DSM-III criteria of self-damaging acts and inappropriate anger predict better results. However, the relationship was weak, and it has not been replicated in other studies.

Some researchers have looked for relationships between early development and outcome. Our group (Paris et al. 1988) reported a correlation between a chart review–derived index of problems with mothers during childhood and lower outcome scores. Stone (1990) described a relationship between "parental brutality" and outcome, but this measure accounted for only 7% of the variance. In a different sample (Paris et al. 1995), we compared a group of women who had recovered from BPD with those who had not and found that childhood sexual abuse was more frequent in those who remained symptomatic compared with a recovered group of the same age. However, because none of these findings was strong, it is unclear whether they have practical significance.

We also lack clinically useful predictors for suicide in patients with BPD. This is troubling but not surprising. Completed suicides are rare events and are always difficult to predict, even in very large samples (Pokorny 1983). Clinicians constantly deal with false positives. Patients with BPD often threaten suicide, yet most never carry it out. (Our anxiety about completion is driven by the minority who die of suicide, patients we never forget.)

Stone found that patients with BPD and substance abuse were more likely to complete suicide. This makes sense because substance abuse itself carries an increased risk (Flavin et al. 1990). Another consistent finding in suicide research is a relationship between number of previous attempts and completion (Maris 2002). Our group (Paris et al. 1989) found that the number of previous attempts in patients with BPD predicted later completion. This result was later confirmed by two Scandinavian studies: a follow-up study of patients treated in an Oslo clinic (Kjeslberg et al. 1994) and a short-term follow-up study comparing patients who suicided within a month of hospitalization with those who did not (Kullgren 1988).

Again, because most multiple attempters never complete suicide, using previous attempts as a criterion leaves us with too many false positives. Moreover, predicting suicide on the basis of past attempts can lead to unnecessary interventions. Chapter 8 suggests that it is futile and counterproductive to respond with alarm to every suicidal thought and gesture in patients with BPD.

In our sample, patients with higher education were statistically more likely to complete suicide (Paris et al. 1988). These results resembled those described by Drake and Gates (1984) for schizophrenia, in which higher social class and high expectations were associated with completion. However, our findings were not replicated in the Oslo study (Kjelsberg et al. 1991). Instead, Kjelsberg's group reported that patients with BPD who experienced separation or loss early in life were more likely to complete suicide, and a similar observation emerged from a psychological autopsy study of young males with BPD who completed suicide (Lesage et al. 1994). Yet none of these developmental variables explains enough of the outcome variance to be of clinical value in predicting fatal outcomes.

In summary, we do not know enough at this point to predict the outcome of BPD, or whether patients will live or die. Some do better than others, but by and large, we really do not know why. To answer this question, it would be useful to understand the mechanisms that mediate recovery. That is the subject of Chapter 7.

Prospective Research

Prospective studies have important advantages for determining the outcome of BPD. When research starts from scratch, baseline data are more reliable, allowing for more accurate identification of clinical predictors. The main limitation of the prospective method is that patients with BPD who agree to be monitored over time may have unique characteristics, such as higher compliance, making them different from the population seen by clinicians.

The other problem with prospective research is expense. Some investigators have begun these projects and then run out of money. Thus far, the most important results have emerged from a study conducted by Paul Links's group at McMaster University in Hamilton, Ontario. Links et al. (1995, 1998) collected a cohort of 130 former inpatients, 88 of whom had a diagnosis of BPD and 42 of whom had only "borderline traits." At the follow-up point, there was some attrition, with 41 subjects not located. The authors found that 2 had died of natural causes, whereas 6 had committed suicide (giving a 7-year completion rate of 5%). In all, 81 patients, of whom 57 had originally met criteria for BPD, were reexamined after 7 years.

The main limitation of this otherwise unique study was that 7 years is not quite long enough to observe the burnout of BPD. This is a phenomenon that usually kicks in between the 10- and 15-year points. There might also have been additional suicides if the cohort had been followed for longer.

Links and colleagues found that about half of the subjects still met criteria for BPD, whereas the other half showed symptomatic recovery. Severity of initial pathology was the best predictor for remission at follow-up evaluation, accounting for 17% of the variance. Links et al. (1995) also compared a subgroup of patients with BPD (about one-quarter of the sample) with those without substance abuse and found that the abusers had a poorer outcome on almost every measure.

More prospective data are needed on the outcome of patients with BPD. Reassessment of the Links et al. cohort after another 7 years would certainly add to our knowledge. However, there are some other current studies that will shed light on the unanswered questions. Zanarini et al. (1998) have been following a cohort previously admitted to McLean Hospital for more than 5 years and will eventually have data on long-term outcome. Their most recent report from the cohort (Zanarini et al. 2003) indicated that the majority of patients with BPD have remissions of their illness and that many recover as early as 6 years after admission. At the same time, several northeastern university sites (Columbia, Harvard, Brown, and Yale) are conducting the NIMH Collaborative Study of Personality Disorders (Gunderson et al. 2000). This research, still in its early stages, has begun tracking a group of patients with BPD, observing the disorder's waxing and waning course (Grilo et al. 2000). The fact that borderline symptoms wax and wane over time may also be one reason why these patients do not always remain in treatment. Similar considerations may apply to other Cluster B categories. We should not think of impulsive personality disorders as having to be present at every cross-sectional follow-up evaluation. Instead, patients can have both good and bad periods, with symptoms reflecting stressful life events.

Prospective studies often use the availability of long-term treatment as a strategy to reduce attrition. Again, the problem is that patients who remain in treatment could be atypical of the larger population with BPD, who typically move in and out of therapy over time (see Chapter) 8. Another knotty problem is how to distinguish between treatment effects and naturalistic recovery.

A 27-Year Outcome Study of Borderline Personality Disorder

Our group has recently conducted a much longer follow-up study of BPD, comparable with the time scale of Black's group in ASPD (Paris and Zweig-Frank 2001). We were primarily interested in finding out whether burnout of borderline pathology continues in later middle age or whether, as McGlashan feared, patients remain vulnerable and again become symptomatic.

In the Introduction, I described the problems we had in obtaining grant support for a project following patients so many years after initial treatment. In the end, we did much better than expected, obtaining information on 81 of the original cohort of 100. Eight patients had died in the intervening years: Five died from natural causes, and there were three additional suicides. Nine patients either failed to answer our letter or refused to talk to us. However, because these subjects had been contacted through the Canadian government, we knew they were still alive. The cohort eventually included 64 individuals (12 men and 52 women), with a mean age of 51 years. The interviews were conducted in 1999, 12 years after the original study, for a mean follow-up time from first admission of 27 years.

We observed a wide range of outcomes, ranging from complete recovery to continued dysfunction. (See Chapter 6 for some detailed clinical examples of these scenarios.) The mean global outcome score was 63, with a standard deviation of 13, the same as we had found 12 years earlier. (These numbers should not be taken too literally, because differences of 5–10 points can easily occur without being truly meaningful—they depend on the rater and on the quality of data used to make the rating.)

Three additional suicides raised the overall rate of completion in the original sample to 10%. The mean age at death was 37.3 ± 10.3 years. (Chapter 9 discusses the significance of this relatively late age of suicide.) The relative male predominance in suicide that we had seen in 1986 was no longer apparent because all of the additional suicides involved women. In total, 6 of our suicides (35%) were male and 11 (65%) were female.

Our cohort showed an unusually high rate of early death. In total, 18.2% of the original sample of 165 patients have died, either from natural causes or from suicide. Applying government statistics (Statistics Canada 1990), we found that the rate was much higher than would be expected for a population of this age. All but 1 of these early deaths involved women. However, there was no pattern for cause of death. The most common fatalities in our group involved cancer or cardiovascular disease; there were also 3 accidental deaths in which there was no evidence of suicidal intent. (One can speculate that a lifetime of impulsivity and affective lability must take its toll on the body.) We were unable to find any consistent predictors of suicide or early death.

The most striking change between 15 and 25 years was the number of subjects who could still be found to have BPD. Only 5 (8% of the total) still met criteria at 27 years, much less than at the 15-year point. At the same time, only 5% had current substance abuse or major depression. The main indicator of continued problems in this sample was that 22% met criteria for dysthymia. This observation may support the theory that affective lability is a core component of BPD, a feature less likely than impulsivity to change over time.

The overall results showed that in spite of great heterogeneity of outcome, at 27-year follow-up evaluation most patients were functioning even better than at 15 years. We also obtained data from a series of self-report questionnaires to assess functioning in more detail: the Hopkins Symptom Check List (Derogatis 1994) and the Social Adjustment Scale (Weissman 1993). These measures, augmented by GAF scores, suggested that symptom levels, as well as levels of social adjustment, were close to normative values for this cohort. Yet qualitatively, the interviews demonstrated residual difficulties in some patients as they grew older, an observation reflected in our quantitative findings on dysthymia.

We then examined our data to determine whether we could identify predictors of 27-year outcome (Zweig-Frank and Paris 2002). Comparing measures at three time periods (baseline, 15 years, and 25 years), we examined whether earlier levels of functioning were significant predictors of later levels. Given the similarity of our subjects at baseline, the DIB-R scores drawn from the chart review were too similar to be predictive of outcome. However, DIB-R scores at 15 years, as well as the GAF scores from that time, were both significant predictors of DIB-R score and GAF score at 27 years. Thus, as is the case for serious mental disorders such as schizophrenia (see Chapter 1), long-term outcome is a function of illness severity. By and large, those who were doing well continued to do well and those who were doing poorly continued to do poorly.

Finally, we examined whether the quality of childhood experiences, as recollected by our subjects, had a relationship to outcome. We administered two self-report questionnaires, the Parental Bonding Index (PBI;

Parker 1983) and the Developmental Experiences Questionnaire (DEQ; Steiger and Zanko 1990). These retrospective instruments are, of course, subject to recall bias, and we have no way of knowing whether they provide an accurate picture of events occurring decades previously.

In any case, no significant findings emerged: None of the PBI scales or the DEQ scales had any relationship to outcome. Thus, patients did as well, or as badly, as would have been expected on the basis of other predictors, independently of how they remembered their childhood. It is possible that characteristics intrinsic to patients with personality disorders are more important in the long run than the quality of early experiences.

Nonetheless, these analyses showed that scores for childhood trauma were remarkably similar to those observed in our studies of younger patients with BPD (Paris et al. 1994a). Over one-third of this sample reported physical and sexual abuse during childhood. These findings, in a middle-aged cohort, were not likely to have reflected recent publicity in the media about childhood trauma and thus support the conclusion that early adversity is a risk factor for BPD.

The PBI findings concerning memories of relationships with parents were surprising in a different way. On the neglect scale, unlike younger samples (Zweig-Frank and Paris 1991), this cohort remembered their parents as having been reasonably affectionate, with scores that did not differ from community norms. It is possible that as patients grow older, childhood memories and perceptions of parents gradually become more mellow. However, on the other PBI scale (parental control), patients with BPD in this older group remembered their parents as more controlling than did younger cohorts. These findings are difficult to explain and may reflect problems in the validity of retrospective measures of parenting.

In summary, our 27-year follow-up study shows that patients with BPD continue to experience improved functionality into their 50s. Over time, most seem to learn to compensate for the problems they experienced when young. In particular, serious impulsivity becomes a thing of the past. However, some continue to have difficulties in intimate relationships that keep them fragile and vulnerable. We look at examples of these issues in Chapter 6.

Commonalities in Outcome Between Antisocial Personality Disorder and Borderline Personality Disorder

Different categories of personality disorders can share underlying commonalities on the trait level. Chapter 2 noted strong similarities in phenomenology and risk factors between ASPD and BPD. The data reviewed in this chapter show that both forms of disorder have remarkably similar outcomes.

Declines in Impulsivity

Patients with ASPD and those with BPD both demonstrate changes in impulsive behavior over time. Patients with ASPD are less likely to get arrested, reduce their use of substances, and are less frequently involved in fraudulent activities. Patients with BPD are less likely to cut themselves or to overdose, and their relationships become less chaotic. Substance abuse also plays a role in predicting outcome in both ASPD and BPD. Those who stop drinking or taking drugs are more likely to do well. Those who continue to use substances either die young or remain disabled.

Continuation of Interpersonal Difficulties

Many patients with ASPD or BPD continue to face serious difficulties in interpersonal relationships, and only some achieve stable intimacy. Patients with ASPD are somewhat more likely to marry and have children but rarely find stable social roles. Patients with BPD may continue to exercise poor judgment about their partners, sometimes giving up on intimacy entirely. Over time, the pathology associated with impulsive personality disorders leads to multiple episodes in which relationships fail. Eventually, one can decide to stop banging one's head against this particular wall. For this reason, the choice to live alone can often be the right one.

Outcome of Other Personality Disorders

Most of the systematic research on long-term outcome has been limited to ASPD and BPD. This situation may change as the NIMH longitudinal study, which also includes patients with disorders in the schizotypal, avoidant, and compulsive categories, collects data. At this point, information on the outcome of other categories described on Axis II is limited to a handful of studies, supplemented by indirect inferences from epidemiological data as well as by clinical reports.

Cluster A Disorders

Most of the existing studies of Cluster A disorders focus on schizotypal personality disorder (SZPD), with minimal data on schizoid personality and none on paranoid personality.

The best study thus far (McGlashan 1986b) followed 10 patients with SZPD who had been hospitalized at Chestnut Lodge. (There were also 18 patients in the follow-up cohort who met criteria for both SZPD and BPD, but these are best considered as predominantly having BPD.) At 15-year follow-up evaluation, this cohort was doing notably more poorly than those with BPD. Only 1 had suicided, but the mean GAF score for the sample was only 49: One-half of the subjects were unemployed, and they had fewer relationships than those with BPD. There were no significant differences between SZPD and schizophrenia, but only 1 subject eventually developed schizophrenia. The others avoided crossing the boundary, surviving on the fringes of society.

The 14-year follow-up study, conducted by Plakun et al. (1985), of patients from Austen Riggs included 13 with SZPD, as well as 19 with schizoid personality disorder. Both groups had improved functionality, with the mean GAF score for the SZPD group being 61 (higher than reported by McGlashan), and with the group with schizoid personality disorder attaining a mean of 67. However, this study was limited by using questionnaires as opposed to interviews, with a minority of patients actually traced.

McGlashan's findings seem more representative of clinical reality. They are also consistent with other data suggesting that patients with Cluster A disorders do not change over time. One line of evidence emerged from a community study (Reich et al. 1989) of personality disorders. When a screening questionnaire was used, Cluster A disorders showed no age cohort effect (i.e., they were just as common later in life as earlier), whereas Cluster B disorders showed a striking falloff in prevalence with age. A recent British community study (Seivewright et al. 2002) also found that patients in Cluster A did not show improved functionality by the time of 12-year follow-up evaluation.

Other Cluster B Disorders

Do histrionic personality disorder (HPD) and narcissistic personality disorder (NPD) follow the same pattern of gradual improvement over time seen in ASPD and BPD? No long-term outcome studies exist for either category, and I am forced to rely on clinical and cross-sectional data.

In the case of HPD, people who are overly flirtatious and dramatic in their youth may need to find another way to remain "the center of attention" as they age. One possibility is that psychopathology might increasingly be expressed through somatic complaints rather than through behavioral patterns. In one study of depressed outpatients (Demopoulos et al. 1996), HPD was associated with increased levels of hypochondriacal concerns. In another study (Apt and Hurlbert 1994), patients with HPD had a higher frequency of sexual problems than did matched control subjects.

Another possibility is that patients with HPD become less flamboyant but continue to have difficulties with intimacy. With time, beauty fades and flirtation drops out of their repertoire. Yet these patients may continue to be emotionally needy, and they lack the skills required to reinvest in less conflictual relationships. These issues must be explored by conducting a formal follow-up study of patients with HPD.

In the case of NPD, we have a small amount of outcome data. Plakun (1991) followed a formerly hospitalized sample of 17 patients for 14 years and found the mean GAF score at outcome to be 65. However, this group could not have been fully representative of the patients with NPD whom most therapists see, in that they required inpatient treatment. We also do not know whether this cohort continued to meet diagnostic criteria at follow-up evaluation.

After a much shorter follow-up period (3 years), Ronningstam (1998) re-evaluated 28 patients with NPD who had been admitted to McLean Hospital. Twenty-eight showed a decline in narcissistic traits, whereas 8 still met criteria for NPD. (This group had more severe difficulties at baseline.) The researchers noted that pathological narcissism can be corrected by life events, ranging from successful achievements to satisfactory relationships. Yet if that is so, we are not really talking about a personality disorder. It is also possible that narcissism waxes and wanes, so that difficulties might reemerge with a longer follow-up period. However, these results can be applied only to patients with severe depression (which would explain why they were hospitalized), which is not the group that psychotherapists often see. I also find it difficult to reconcile the findings of Ronningstam with my clinical experience, which is that patients with NPD are unusually resistant to change.

Kernberg (1976), drawing on his long clinical experience with patients with NPD, suggested that because narcissism eventually declines with age, some patients become treatable only in later life. Kernberg argued that when people are very young, the social environment tends to reinforce grandiosity and to encourage externalization, and that these reinforcements interfere with the therapeutic process. In contrast, as people grow older, disappointments leading to a deflated and depleted sense of self become inevitable, eliciting sufficient depressive feelings to make introspection possible. Although I find these ideas clinically appealing, I await systematic data to confirm them.

Cluster C Disorders

There are few systematic data on the long-term outcome of patients with Cluster C disorders, but indirect evidence suggests that avoidant, dependent, and compulsive personality structures tend to remain stable over time. The community study conducted by Reich et al. (1989) had found no age cohort effect for Cluster C disorders. In other words, older people were just as likely as younger people to present with similar difficulties, in contrast to the outcome for Cluster B disorders.

Recent data from a community study from a primary care sample in England (Seivewright et al. 2002; Tyrer and Seivewright 2000) sheds further light on the outcome for patients with Cluster C disorders. This study found that patients with Cluster C personality disorders did not have improved functionality by 12-year follow-up evaluation. Moreover, certain traits characteristic of this group (anxiousness, vulnerability, conscientiousness) increased over time. Many withdrew increasingly from human relationships and became more symptomatic and dysphoric. As they aged, these patients experienced increasing isolation and lack of social support and developed Axis I symptomatology (largely mood and anxiety disorders).

Summary

Most patients with ASPD do poorly, but the outcome for those with BPD is more unpredictable. The findings can be divided into the proverbial good news and bad news: Although most patients have improved functionality, many continue to show some degree of impairment and many die prematurely, either from natural causes or from suicide. Yet some patients with the most severe pathology eventually recover with time; although one might think that those with the worst pathology suicide or die early, there is no predictable relationship between severity and fatality.

In contrast, other personality disorders tend to remain chronic. Patients with Cluster A disorders are disabled by the negative symptoms their disorders share with schizophrenia, and they lack the positive symptoms that tend to remit. Patients with Cluster C disorders have anxiety traits that can be self-reinforcing over time, characteristics that may not improve with age.

6

Patients With Borderline Personality Disorder After 27 Years

This chapter presents 16 clinical examples, which comprise one-quarter of the sample I interviewed in 1999 for our 27-year follow-up study of patients with borderline personality disorder (BPD). Paralleling the gender distribution of the group, I describe here 14 women and 2 men. Identifying details have been changed to protect the confidentiality of the participants.

The cohort can usefully be considered in five groups:

A. Two cases of patients who still met criteria for BPD.
B. Two cases of patients whose functioning remained marginal, even though symptoms fell below the diagnostic threshold.
C. Five cases of patients whose functioning improved but who retained clinically significant symptoms, each with a different pathway to remission.
D. Four cases of patients with no residual symptoms, each with a unique pathway to recovery.
E. Three cases of patients who completed suicide, pointing to reasons for fatal outcomes.

Group A: Still Meeting Criteria for Borderline Personality Disorder

Case 1

In her 20s, Frances was one of the most "famous" patients with BPD treated at our hospital. Constantly in and out of the ward or the emergency holding area, she had more than 20 admissions. All of these hospitalizations followed suicidal threats or overdoses, and Frances was also a chronic self-cutter. She was best known for her violent rages, some of which led to physical attacks on staff members.

Frances had been a severe alcoholic for many years and became promiscuously involved with a series of unstable men. Frances lacked stability anywhere in her life: She had a ninth-grade education and had never been able to hold a steady job.

At 27-year follow-up evaluation, Frances, then 49, was functioning on a low level. As she aged, her life came to center more and more on the hospital clinic, and her social network consisted of other patients she met there. She was unemployed and living alone, with few interests and no family support.

Frances complained of chronic depression, panic attacks, and suicidal thoughts. Although she no longer drank, she was still abusing prescribed benzodiazepines. During the interview, her mood was highly labile, moving in and out of negative affective states.

Frances's last overdose and hospitalization occurred 3 years previously. She had stopped cutting herself 7 years earlier. Her last serious suicide threat had occurred 1 year previously, at which time she threw herself in front of a car when refused admission to hospital. (She was not hurt.) Frances was not in any form of psychotherapy and was being monitored by a family doctor to renew her prescriptions (paroxetine hydrochloride [Paxil] and chlorpromazine). All of her previous therapists refused to see her again, in view of her history of harassment and threats against them—information that was well known in the clinic.

Comments

I have seen hundreds of patients with BPD, but Frances was one of the sickest. She has been a trial and a challenge to many experienced therapists.

In medicine, the most severely ill patients usually have the worst prognosis, and it was not surprising to find Frances to be doing poorly. At the same time, I describe other patients in this chapter who were just as difficult and problematic as Frances and whose outcome was better, some of them finding an occupational niche in spite of limited education. (See "Bill," Case 3, as well as "Mary," Case 6.)

Alternatively, one might ask, given her low quality of life, why Frances never committed suicide (compare "Rachel," Case 13). Many of her attempts had been serious, and Frances had been treated several times in intensive care units. Patients with BPD play Russian roulette with their lives, and overdoses have an unpredictable outcome. Whether suicidal patients live or die may depend on random factors such as whether intended rescuers turn up or the accessibility of effective medical care.

Case 2

Joanne had a series of admissions to hospitals in her 20s, occurring after a series of suicide attempts. Each of these crises was associated with a disappointment in love. Joanne always had trouble with men. She has described her younger self as a beauty and a flower child; she even worked briefly as a stunt double in a film. Over the years, Joanne has almost always been able to hold a job but has never been able to sustain an intimate relationship. She was briefly married in her 30s, and that relationship produced a child.

At the time of follow-up evaluation, Joanne was 50 and temporarily unemployed. She was living with her 16-year-old daughter and her elderly mother. Until just before the follow-up interview, she had held an excellent job as a teacher in a secretarial school. She lost this position when she ran off impulsively to another city to follow a man. At the same time, she burned her bridges by quarreling seriously with her boss. The relationship did not last long, and the new lover quickly dumped her, after which she returned home. At the time of the interview, she was involved with a drug-abusing neighbor, unable to break off with him for fear of loneliness.

In spite of these problems, Joanne had not been in therapy for many years. She was not taking any medication. Her only recent contact with the mental health system had involved a consultation with a social worker concerning problems with her daughter.

Joanne was the only member of our cohort to develop clinical problems after the interview. I had made an initial call from my home, leaving a message on her answering machine. However, I failed to take into account recent technological advances that allowed Joanne to access my private number. For a time she began to call me rather frequently. Fortunately, it was easy to get her to stop this behavior by informing her that she was being disruptive, and that if she continued I would be too upset to arrange further help. (I also learned how to use the blocking code on my phone.)

I referred Joanne to a psychologist on our crisis team who had extensive experience in cognitive therapy. The therapy turned out to be stormy. Joanne would call me (at work) to complain about the fact that she was being strongly encouraged to get herself another job. Nonetheless, she did complete a 3-month course of treatment. After discharge, she obtained a new job as a receptionist, and she has not recontacted our clinic.

Comments

Personality disorders have a waxing and waning course. Thus, even if patients do not score as having BPD in any specific month, the chronic course of pathology becomes apparent over a longer period. Joanne had scored positive for BPD at the 15-year point, but her work history was superior to some in our cohort who scored negative. As it happened, the 27-year follow-up interview caught her during a serious crisis.

Throughout her life, Joanne had been heavily invested in her physical appearance. As a result, aging became a major problem, leading her to feel desperate about her future. Although Joanne had been able to attain some stability by working, she has lacked steadiness and commitment. Her difficulties as a parent relate to problems in putting the needs of a child before her own, difficulties that are not, in my experience, unusual among patients with BPD.

Group B: No Longer Having Borderline Personality Disorder but Functioning at a Marginal Level

Case 3

Bill was another of our "famous" patients—residents would often wonder if he was going to turn up when they were assigned night call. Starting in late adolescence, he had been hospitalized on many occasions after overdoses or suicidal threats.

On one occasion, when I saw Bill in the emergency department around midnight, he responded to my reluctance to admit him by walking to a sink and taking out his bottle of medication with the intention to swallow it all. I responded, instinctively, by knocking the bottle out of his hands, and sending pills flying all over the room. This was hardly the way to convince a patient to go home. Bill won that particular power struggle, and he spent that night in hospital.

Bill was also known for violent rages and often had to be put into restraints. Although peripherally involved in the drug culture, he rarely turned up under the influence. Instead, he usually came to the hospital after disappointments in relationships. Bill had only brief and unsatisfactory liaisons with women and had never achieved long-term intimacy. His instability was further fueled by the fact that he had not finished high school and had never attained stable employment.

As is often the case with patients with BPD (even more so when they are men), Bill's diagnosis was questioned by the staff. The most confusing point was that he often presented with "paranoid" ideas (e.g., that someone in his apartment house had it in for him). However, these thoughts were exaggerations of real situations and were never bizarre. More confusingly (at least for those unfamiliar with the frequency of micropsychotic symptoms in

BPD), Bill intermittently heard critical voices in his head. Although these symptoms appeared only when he was stressed, he was treated for psychosis over many years with injectable antipsychotic medication. Bill actually liked attending this clinic and getting injections. It gave him a reason to come in every 2 weeks and to talk about his life with a nurse. He also sought out psychotherapy for his interpersonal problems, at one point even paying for a psychologist's services privately out of his welfare allowance.

At the age of 44, Bill was living in a supervised apartment project administrated by the hospital. He was making additional money by cooking meals for other people in his building. He also sold goods (possibly stolen) in a secondhand market, calling this project his "business." All of these settings provided him with a social network that did not require intimacy. Although he still has occasional flings with women, there has been nothing serious. He maintains no contact with his family, even though two sisters live in the same town where he does.

Bill had recently been feeling more optimistic and energetic. He had not thought of suicide for a long time, no longer hears voices, and had no paranoid ideas. Moreover, Bill has not been hospitalized in the last 10 years. Although he still attends our clinic and makes use of a subsidized housing program, his contact has become limited to refilling his medications (now oral)—risperidone and carbamazepine (Tegretol).

Comments

Bill will probably be a lifelong patient, but he no longer presents serious clinical problems. Having survived the worst of his illness, Bill reached a point in life where remission set in.

In light of my previous contact with him, the extent of his recovery came as a bit of a surprise. In his 20s and 30s, in spite of a vast investment of treatment resources, nothing we did seemed to help. Yet after turning 40, he became less aggressive, less impulsive, less depressed—even less "psychotic." It seems unlikely that changing his neuroleptics from typicals to atypicals was helpful; it is also possible that, as was the case for others in our sample, his psychotic symptoms might have remitted without risperidone. (This hypothesis is hard to test, because his psychiatrists remain understandably reluctant to discontinue his medication.)

Case 4

Leila was first admitted to our hospital at age 23 after a serious overdose. In the 1960s she had been deeply involved in the drug culture, using hashish, alcohol, and cocaine on a regular basis.

Leila had a tenth-grade education and has always worked as a waitress. She had a daughter out of wedlock at 28 and was married for 7 years in her 30s. This relationship ended 15 years ago under dramatic circumstances— her daughter informed her that the stepfather had been molesting her, and she left him the same day. This incident had a deep resonance for Leila. She had grown up in a dysfunctional family, raised by an alcoholic father and a depressed mother. Between the ages of 5 and 6 years, Leila was sexually abused by an uncle, but she told me that she was so starved for love that she actually missed him when he disappeared from her life.

Five years ago, Leila joined Narcotics Anonymous, and she has been clean ever since. She describes Narcotics Anonymous as her "fellowship"— it provides her with a sponsor and a social network. Leila has seen several psychologists for therapy and was also in primal therapy shortly after the breakup of her marriage. Recently she has been taking courses in massage therapy but finds this a difficult project and thinks of quitting.

Leila is now 52. She works part time as a waitress. Leila has few friends and feels quite lonely: She has not been with a man since she left her husband and is also estranged from her daughter. Yet Leila is in good health, other than chronic insomnia and intermittent feelings of depression. She takes no medications, largely because of past drug problems. Leila has not self-mutilated since she was a teenager. However, she still hears voices in her head—a "committee" that makes negative comments. Leila also describes frequent episodes of depersonalization, feeling physically and mentally estranged from the world. Leila expressed the wish that the rest of her life could somehow make up for some of what she missed in the first 50 years.

Comments

If I had interviewed Leila a few years previously, she would probably have still met criteria for BPD. Now a marked decline in impulsivity has moved her out of this category. Nonetheless, given the level of her problems, I would diagnose her pathology by DSM-IV-TR (American Psychiatric Association 2000) as personality disorder not otherwise specified. The continued presence of micropsychotic symptoms is unusual; these features tend to remit with time. To the extent that hallucinatory phenomena in BPD are mood-related, Leila's level of chronic dysphoria might have been high enough to stoke her cognitive symptoms.

The most important factor in Leila's remission involved giving up drugs. As described earlier in the book, many substance abusers recover in middle age. In this case, as in so many others, a key factor in maintaining stability was membership in an "anonymous" support group.

Group C: Clinically Improved but With Residual Symptoms

Case 5

Penny had multiple hospitalizations for cutting, suicide attempts, and drug abuse. I had known her when I was a resident in psychiatry, and she was one of the most colorful characters on the ward. Intelligent, eloquent, and sardonic in manner, she made a distinct impression on everyone she met. At that time, Penny was married, and she and her husband were in charge of a foster home for disturbed children. The marriage ended a few years later, after which Penny then moved to Western Canada; there were no children. Since her divorce, she has been exclusively gay and has had a serious of lesbian relationships.

Penny had just turned 50 when I interviewed her. She told me, "I didn't expect to live that long." Penny has made no further suicide attempts in the last 15 years, even though she sometimes thinks about suicide as a possibility. At present her drug use is confined to daily marijuana. Penny no longer wants to get overly attached to anyone and states that breakups are "learning experiences." A recent relationship ended a few months ago, and Penny lives alone in a small apartment. She has been estranged for many years from her mother as well as from all her siblings.

Penny has become a television producer, with several documentaries about the mentally ill to her credit. In this way, she has been able to turn her own experiences (and an acute capacity for observation) into a successful career. She also works part time as a patient advocate.

Penny told me she converted her own personal disappointment with psychiatric care into a mission. She also enjoys the attention her work has brought her; people on the street sometimes notice her (although she admits this is most likely due to her unusual hats).

Comments

Penny's good outcome was associated with talents she learned to put to good use. She benefits from public attention and has turned borderline rage into effective advocacy.

Penny's residual difficulties were largely related to an inability to establish stable intimate relationships. Initially, Penny had been firmly heterosexual, and her later turn to homosexuality might have been an attempt to deal with her chronic disappointments with men. Yet given her powerful needs and her dominating personality, it is not entirely surprising that Penny had similar difficulties managing intimacy with women.

Case 6

Mary had been another "famous" patient at our hospital. Her many hospitalizations almost always resulted from overdoses of medication. Mary had also spent time in jail—for shoplifting and for assault. Because of her violent rages, she was "blacklisted" from the emergency department and clinic for several years. In 1987, after learning that Mary had been invited by my team to participate in the 15-year follow-up evaluation, the director of emergency services was quite angry.

Mary was the third of 13 children, and she reported that her mother was unable to cope with the burden, using physical punishment freely as a method of control. Fortunately, Mary was an intelligent girl who attained consistent success in school; she eventually completed a master's degree in special education. Even at the peak of her difficulties, she worked as a teacher of retarded children. At the time, I found it striking that someone who functioned in a responsible job by day could come night after night to the emergency department and behave in such a regressed fashion.

I had last seen Mary 12 years ago, at which time she was doing poorly, having even given up her job. All of her relationships with men had been short-term and unsuccessful, and she was becoming increasingly isolated.

I was therefore very surprised to find her nearly asymptomatic at age 50. The reason for her recovery came as an even greater surprise. In her late 30s, Mary had gone to see a psychiatrist, with whom she fell in love. The therapist was a man 15 years her senior, and he returned her feelings, eventually leaving his wife and children for her. To avoid scandal, the couple moved to a rural area in another province. At the time of follow-up evaluation, they had been together for 11 years, without children, and had finally "made it official" 2 years previously. They remain almost completely involved with each other, to the exclusion of a social network.

The main problem at present for Mary is her husband's health. He developed lung cancer with brain metastases 2 years ago but was in remission after a course of radiotherapy. The husband plans to retire soon, after which they might move back to Montreal. Mary has not held a job of her own since she moved away, and she attributes this to her "chronic fatigue syndrome." (In spite of this condition, she described herself as full of energy.)

Mary's main current symptom is chronic insomnia, which she has had all her life, and for which she occasionally needs diazepam (Valium). She has not attempted suicide or cut herself in 12 years, although she occasionally thinks about it. Mary also continues to seek out occasional therapy, recently attending a support program in another city designed for trauma victims.

Comments

Mary's recovery was a big surprise, but in retrospect, it can be seen that there had been some positive prognostic signs. In spite of a deprived background, she had obtained postgraduate training and developed a successful professional career. The same persistence led her from therapy to therapy in constant hope of improvement.

As Gutheil (1992) has pointed out, patients with BPD are particularly likely to become sexually involved with professionals who treat them (assuming, of course, that the therapists agree). Usually, this leads to disaster, and most jurisdictions now suspend or remove the license of any therapist who allows such a scenario to unfold. Although the outcome in this case was positive, it is highly exceptional, and one would hardly recommend this method of recovery to other patients with BPD.

However, these patients require a holding environment, and marriage may be one way to meet that need, particularly if they have been previously stabilized by a relationship with a psychotherapist. My own experience has been that some patients with BPD have improved functionality after marriage and that others do not. The question is what determines outcome. Personal characteristics of the spouse may be a factor (Paris and Braverman 1995). For example, a man with narcissistic personality disorder may choose a woman with BPD because she is totally devoted to him. Relationships of this kind are inherently unstable. The particular combination of narcissistic and borderline pathology creates an explosive mixture that is usually fatal to marriage. Alternatively, a man who is emotionally constrained may be attracted to a woman with BPD who seems vibrantly emotional. This scenario also has its dangers, particularly if the husband responds to his wife's excessive demands by withdrawal. On the other hand, a husband who is a steady and reliable presence might help a woman with BPD to modulate her affective instability.

Mary has done well in a kind of symbiotic marriage. However, with a husband who is in poor health, she may soon have to manage widowhood, and it is difficult to predict how she will cope with that role.

Case 7

Florence had her first hospitalization at age 19 years as a nursing student, followed by additional admissions over the course of her 20s. Florence was an alcoholic who drank to combat her mood instability. She would also cut herself and/or take overdoses when intimate relationships did not work out. An early marriage quickly broke up, and she had no children.

Florence had 9 years of therapy with a psychiatrist at our hospital who saw her twice a week and prescribed disulfiram (Antabuse) for her. This treatment kept her out of hospitals but had little impact on her interpersonal difficulties. Therapy ended when she became involved with a boyfriend who was moving to another city and she followed him to Europe. When the relationship broke up, Florence was suicidal, leading to another admission. Rapidly pulling herself together, Florence became more involved in her work, training herself to be a specialist in an oncology clinic.

At 56, Florence is working as a nurse in an outpatient clinic. She states she likes her job because it provides contact with people. Florence has had no intimate relations with men for 10 years. Her social life has become increasingly limited, much of it centering around Alcoholics Anonymous, and her best friends are her two cats. She remains on good terms with her ex-boyfriend, who still visits her on a platonic basis, even though he has since married another woman.

Florence has been abstinent from alcohol for 10 years. She began taking sertraline (Zoloft) 4 years ago and thinks she becomes more depressed if she reduces the dose. At the time of the interview, she was sleeping well and had a good deal of energy.

Florence is a personable woman who asked to be interviewed face-to-face. In spite of a reserved manner, she ended our meeting by asking, "So, do we have another date in 10 years?"

Comments

Florence's recovery demonstrates several important points about the outcome of BPD. First, recovery is associated with an ability to control substance abuse. Second, she maintained a job, and a sense of accomplishment at work can function as a "reserve tank" of self-esteem, even when interpersonal relationships turn out to be messy and painful. Finally, Florence is one of many patients with BPD who found that avoiding intimacy removed them from the arena where their most serious problems occurred.

Case 8

Carol had dealt with drug abuse, mood instability, suicide attempts, and a series of unsatisfactory relationships with men. Carol was unhappy with all of her psychiatrists and usually broke off treatment with them within a few months.

Carol stopped using drugs in her early 30s, and she married at age 38 years. This relationship has stabilized her. She is very dependent on her husband and has had no children. She also remains close to her two identical sisters, Joan and Ilene. The triplets had all had serious difficulties after the divorce of their parents—all three required therapy, and all three met criteria for BPD. Joan had been hospitalized for suicidality and an eating disorder. She went on to have four children and seems to be stable in a second marriage. Ilene was also suicidal in her 20s but recovered after giving up drugs. She became a legal secretary, is married with no children, but is undergoing long-term antidepressant therapy. Interestingly, all three were brought up as Jewish and converted to Christianity, remaining active in Protestant churches.

At 47, Carol is doing better. She has been working for the federal government for the past 13 years, and her husband works in the same office. She described some sense of fragility, fearing "another breakdown." Carol has been in therapy with the same social worker for the last 4 years. She finds this contact necessary and has no plans to terminate. Carol has also been taking pimozide since 1984, although she could not explain exactly why. (She denied having had psychotic symptoms.) Since 1995, when she began to experience more depression, she has also been taking paroxetine hydrochloride (Paxil).

Comments

Carol was of particular interest to me because she was one of a group of identical triplets who had all been treated at our hospital and had all been scored by me as having BPD in the chart review. I would have liked to have interviewed all of them to document phenotypical differences between three women with the same genotype (in parallel with the "Genain quadruplets," the schizophrenic women described in Chapter 1). However, at both follow-up points, Carol was the only one of the three we could interview.

Carol demonstrates two mechanisms of improvement in BPD. A successful marriage can help stabilize the disorder by damping down impulsivity. Religious conversion can also be helpful to patients with BPD, by providing a connection with a benevolent deity and by establishing links with a supportive community united in a common belief.

Case 9

Suzanne tells the story of a horrific childhood. Her mother, who also seemed to suffer from BPD (with many suicide attempts throughout her life) was a drug addict, and her father was a military man diagnosed as a "psychopath." The father sexually abused several of his seven children, including Suzanne, who was the oldest. To escape this highly dysfunctional family, Suzanne married young and then gave birth to four children of her own.

Her first admission to the hospital occurred at age 20 years, after her first child was born. For many years thereafter, she was chronically suicidal. Suzanne also heard voices arguing in her head and at times even felt as if she were developing several personalities, accompanied by frequent feelings of unreality.

At age 46, Suzanne has been on her own for 9 years. Suzanne is no longer in therapy and takes no medications. Her marriage ended in divorce, and she never remarried. Suzanne has worked on a volunteer basis in a shelter for abused women and eventually went back to school. She works as an administrative assistant in the same university where she is a student and has just managed to complete an honors degree in psychology. Thus, after a difficult period, Suzanne's life is on the upswing. However, since her divorce, she has not been seriously involved with another man.

Suzanne joined a Mennonite church (a liberal one) in her area. At first she did not feel she was fitting in, but she gradually became part of the community. Although she attributes her recovery to her own efforts, Suzanne also feels she benefited from a strong relationship to God.

Comments

Suzanne's story reflects some of the most common mechanisms of recovery from BPD. She could not manage intimacy, and learned to avoid it. She developed a career that provided her with a sense of self-esteem that was not dependent on a relationship with another person. She joined a strong religious community that provided her with emotional support that was also independent of intimacy.

Group D: No Residual Symptoms

Case 10

Marianne was one of the first patients I treated in psychotherapy during my residency. She was then a 19-year-old nursing student who had complained of depression and was referred by her supervisor to a psychiatrist. He immediately prescribed an antidepressant, but Marianne felt misunderstood and not listened to. She then angrily swallowed the whole bottle, leading to a hospital admission.

Marianne was a lonely young woman in chronic conflict with her family, by whom she also felt deeply misunderstood. When her parents were interviewed, they described her as always having been an "extremist." Her father, a man with a military career, had moved around the country a lot. Her mother, because she was unhappy with this life, was less than responsive to the children. When Marianne was angry with her parents, she would sometimes refuse to communicate with them in French (her native language), speaking to them in English as a dramatic way of showing them her alienation.

Marianne's functioning improved while she was in the hospital, but she also became involved in a symbiotic relationship with another patient with BPD on the ward, who may have played some role in shaping her symptoms. Shortly before her discharge Marianne experienced a micropsychotic episode, with disorientation and auditory hallucinations. This lasted for only 1 day, but she was given a low-dose neuroleptic for several months.

Marianne completed school and took a position in a laboratory, where she quickly rose in the hierarchy. Therapy appeared to be helpful in improving her relationship with her family. She also became involved with a young businessman, and when she married him at age 23, we agreed to end treatment.

Ten years later, Marianne divorced her husband after she had a long-term affair with a married doctor working in her company. She had no children by her husband but became pregnant at age 35 by her lover, making the conscious choice to keep the child. She then separated from her lover and raised their son on her own. Since then there has been no other man in her life, and she does not feel she needs one.

At 49, Marianne has a responsible job at her company, gets to travel a lot, and enjoys her work. She has had no further therapy over the past 25 years. Although Marianne's choices in life were somewhat unconventional, she had no symptoms at follow-up evaluation.

Comments

Marianne's recovery has been stable for many years. Among the positive prognostic factors have been her commitment to and involvement in her career. Intimate relationships have presented more problems for her. She married a man who was solid but not particularly sensitive. After unsuccessfully pursuing him to provide the level of emotional responsiveness she thought she needed, Marianne withdrew from the marriage. Her long-term affair with a married man can be understood in many ways, but one important factor was that she did not have to live with him. Instead, she experienced the excitement of a secret romance without having to bear the disillusionment of intimacy. Similarly, Marianne was more successful as a single mother than as a wife. Unlike some women with BPD who recreate interpersonal conflicts with their children, Marianne found that raising a child avoided her difficulties associated with depending on someone with whom she was intimate.

Case 11

Tom was an adolescent who realized early that he was gay but who had great difficulty coming out. Tom's trouble accepting his identity led to open conflict with his family. He was hospitalized on several occasions for suicide attempts, and his treatment reflected some of the fads of the 1960s. Thus, Tom received a long course of electroconvulsive therapy and was also prescribed aversion therapy to eliminate erotic responses to homosexual imagery (an intervention that he thinks still interferes with sexual functioning). After this period he began to live in the counterculture, experimenting with a number of drugs.

Tom's view is that he improved in spite of rather than because of psychiatric help. Once Tom accepted his sexual orientation, he never again had contact with the mental health system. He moved to another city to put some distance between himself and his family and went into business. By his early 30s, Tom had started his own company. At 51, in spite of having only a tenth-grade education, he was president of a successful firm.

Tom has lived with a series of three stable partners, with some cruising on the side. He is active in the gay rights movement. Tom states that he has a rewarding social life and enjoys traveling and racquetball.

Comments

Tom does not believe he was ever really sick but just had to deal with a homophobic social environment, recovering once he came out. I see the matter a little differently. I have seen a number of patients of this kind over the years. Although the environment of those times was different, very few young men who came out, even 40 years ago, had the kind of difficulties he experienced. Tom, like other patients with BPD, may have had an impulsive and affectively unstable temperament, characteristics that became contained when he established a gay identity. His success in work also provided him with sufficient self-esteem to put his troubles behind him.

Case 12

Nora presented with typical BPD symptoms (suicide, self-mutilation, drugs, unstable relationships). These difficulties lasted until she reached the age of 26. At that point, she converted from Judaism to a fundamentalist form of Christianity. From that point on, she had no further symptoms and has not sought further help.

Nora had an unsuccessful first marriage that ended 10 years ago but feels the divorce was untraumatic because she initiated it and because she had her religious faith. She is now remarried to an active Christian, and they have a 2-year-old child.

At 45, Nora is a practicing social worker. She describes her life as happy and successful, with no symptoms of any kind, and a large circle of friends. In Nora's view, psychiatry did not help her, because she felt blamed rather than validated and because she was given medication that did not help her.

Comments

One of the more intriguing aspects of BPD is the search for meaning. For most of us, existential anxiety is a passing phenomenon with little long-term impact on our lives. For those with BPD, however, the hunger for meaning is as essential as that for food.

Some life choices have the capacity to contain the traits that underlie BPD. Whether this involves developing a gay identity (Case 11) or, as in this case, a religious commitment, the identity diffusion characteristic of BPD can reorganize itself around an external defined identity. This same process has been described in a previous chapter to account for the rare recoveries from antisocial personality disorder, which can be associated with religious conversion.

In a longitudinal study of children at risk, Werner and Smith (1992) noted that fundamentalist religion was a major protective factor against adult psychopathology. In general, religious observances are positively associated with mental health (Koenig 2001). In the recovery process, strong commitments provide relief from symptoms. Thus, many women with BPD who have children become less impulsive, largely because responsibility for the next generation makes suicidal acting out almost unthinkable. Similarly, as demonstrated by several patients in this cohort, commitment to an occupation provides many with sufficient meaning to damp down their impulsivity, at least as long as they are working. Commitment to a cause, either to a political movement or to a religious faith, which also provides powerful bonds to a community, may be even more sustaining over time.

Case 13

I now return to the case (described in Chapter 2) of Ellen, an adolescent who presented with typical symptoms of BPD. Ellen emerged from a highly adverse family environment, with an alcoholic mother and a paranoid, incestuous father. She may, however, have benefited from having been in foster care over several years during early childhood. Her later return to the care of her parents led to her being exposed to severe trauma, from which she was rescued by placement with an older sister.

I treated Ellen for 2 years in psychotherapy. Her course was chaotic and troubled, and she had a psychiatric hospitalization for threatened suicide, as well as a medical hospitalization for an overdose. However, in spite of her chronic suicidality, she continued to do well in school. Ellen benefited from having an engaging personality that always earned her friendship and support from others.

Ellen's impulsivity and problems with dependency expressed themselves in the manner in which she terminated this therapy. She had started a relationship with a new boyfriend and left treatment angrily when I asked questions about why she was getting involved so quickly. Most probably, Ellen felt ready for more autonomy but could not work through a formal termination.

Ellen called me back about 2 years later. She asked me to return to her a large number of letters she had written. In fact, she had written me every day as a way of maintaining contact between sessions. The entire collection of letters was placed in what she called a "Paris file" and was delivered to me shortly before her therapy ended. I was concerned about this request, because I had moved to a different office and had disposed of a great deal of paper, including the Paris file. However, when I explained to Ellen that I no longer had this material, she readily accepted my explanation.

When Ellen was interviewed in 1986, she was 25 years old and living temporarily in another city. By this time, Ellen had already recovered from BPD. She was working and was in a stable marriage (with the same man she had met 6 years before). She attained the highest GAF score (80) of any subject in our 15-year follow-up study.

In 1992, at the age of 31 years, Ellen returned for further treatment with me, which lasted for 18 months. By that time she had two young daughters. She was concerned that she might damage them as her mother had damaged her. If anything, Ellen functioned as a "supermother" whose constant activity was designed to avoid any disaster. Her own mother, still actively alcoholic, was back in her life. Most of the therapeutic work consisted of helping her to establish better boundaries in that relationship. In doing so, she became less anxious about her management of her own family. Ellen also showed resourcefulness in becoming involved in activities outside the family. She worked part-time for a printing company and was also involved in activities at the neighborhood school.

I saw Ellen again in 1996, when she was 35 years old. At this time, therapy focused more on her feelings about men. At this time, her father was dying, and she had borne a third child, this time a son. She was also concerned about her husband, who had been treated for pericarditis and who worried her by heavy use of marijuana.

At the time of the last follow-up interview in 1999, Ellen was 38 years old and happy with her marriage and her children. Her husband had become successful in business, although Ellen continued to be upset about his cannabis dependence. Meanwhile, although her mother continues to drink, she is no longer creating a great deal of trouble. Ellen's main regret at this point is that she has not been able to launch a career. She has a bachelor of arts degree and wants to use her brain, so she might go back to school when her son is in first grade. Ellen experienced no symptoms at all, with the exception of mood swings that she described as being of manageable proportions.

Comments

Although Ellen retained residual problems reflecting her earlier traits of impulsivity and affective instability, her functioning now fell well within normal limits. I would like to take credit for Ellen's recovery. I am even tempted—as I have seen colleagues do about patients with such favorable outcomes—to talk about this patient to the exclusion of all the patients with BPD whom I have treated who had a mediocre or a negative outcome! As a researcher, however, I know that her course was atypical of BPD. The long-term outcome of this case probably has more to do with Ellen than with the treatment she received.

Group E: Suicide Completions—How and Why

Case 14

Rachel was another patient whose emergency-department visits and frequent admissions to hospital had made her "famous" among the staff. From late adolescence onward, Rachel had been in and out of hospitals because of chronic depression, severe anxiety, and continuous suicidal ideas. She also presented with several serious suicide attempts and repeated wrist slashing. Finally, Rachel described intermittent ideas of reference about people in the street, episodes of depersonalization, and visual hallucinations (flashing colored lights) and auditory hallucinations (banging sounds in the head, a female voice criticizing her, a male voice telling her to die). Rachel also had several medical problems, most particularly chronic bowel obstruction, and had once undergone a medical workup to see if she had a demyelinating disease.

Rachel's childhood was unusually deprived. She had been placed in a foster home at age 4 because of her mother's serious child abuse. Her mother had alcoholism, and her father was a criminal who eventually died in a gangland slaying. Her stepfather was a severe gambler, and both he and her mother worked in pornographic movies.

Rachel became a multiple substance abuser by the age 16 years and also sold drugs. She became a prostitute to support these habits. Her one "straight" job was as a dental hygienist for a few years. Later, she was largely unemployed, working intermittently as a stripper and a prostitute. Her other impulsive activities included cocaine and alcohol abuse, as well as gambling. She had lived with several men for months at a time but never married, and she became increasingly socially isolated over the years.

Rachel was doing poorly at the time of her 15-year follow-up interview. She was unemployed and ill and felt she was growing old alone. Rachel had not been helped by therapy and did not see herself as getting any better. Two years later, at age 35 years, she committed suicide by overdose.

Comments

Rachel exemplifies a severe form of BPD. Yet when I last saw her, a year before her death, I thought she might be entering a phase of burnout. She had become much less impulsive and required fewer admissions to hospitals. Perhaps the staff also felt burned out. Like Frances (Case 1), Rachel reached a point at which no therapist at the hospital was willing to treat her. In the last 2 years of her life, she was being seen by a social worker who provided her with some support but who had little time to deal with her complex problems.

Rachel may have decided on suicide at a point when all attempts to help her had failed and she had lost hope for recovery. Alternatively, the final overdose may have been another of her many gambles with death, but this time she was not rescued.

Case 15

Gail is the only patient in the study I knew personally. When I was a psychiatric resident, she lived next door and occasionally baby-sat for my children. Gail was a talented violinist and entertained, at least for a time, thoughts of a serious career, and her family members were ambitious for her. Sitting in the yard, I could often hear her practicing a Mozart concerto.

Gail was described by her parents as a difficult child who would scream for hours and could never be properly comforted. Her parents were immigrants who both worked hard to make a life for themselves in Canada. Unlike her older brother, who readily attained success in all areas, Gail felt like a failure. She was lonely in school, making only the occasional friend. As Gail matured, she remained consistently unsuccessful in achieving intimate relationships and did not seem to trust anyone who came close to her. She was never able to fall in love with a man. Her closest attachment, however conflictual, was always with her mother.

Gail's first hospital admission occurred at age 12 years for anorexia nervosa. She responded to the treatment, but her symptoms later changed to those of bulimia, accompanied by compulsive exercise. The second admission, at age 17 years, occurred after Gail slashed her wrists after severe conflict with her family. At first Gail responded well to psychotherapy. The resident assigned to her case followed her for a year after discharge. She returned to school and continued to have academic success.

After deciding she could not develop into a professional musician, Gail left home and obtained a scholarship to study at an elite university in the United States. She received more therapy while she was there but was not rehospitalized. After graduation, she entered law school in Canada, in a city far from her home.

Gail's life started to fall apart during law school. Although she managed to pass her courses every year, she was in and out of hospitals during this time, with overdoses, wrist slashing, and episodes of self-burning. She had very stormy relationships with her psychiatrists. Gail would either dismiss a therapist for lack of understanding or be herself dismissed. On the last occasion, treatment ended when she threw an ashtray at her psychiatrist, who refused to see her again.

Gail worked for a year after graduation and was then offered a job in a law firm. Shortly before she was scheduled to begin, Gail took a fatal overdose. She was 28 years old.

Comments

Gail was unusual in two ways. First, she was by far the youngest suicide in our sample. Her early despair was probably related to her inability to attain intimacy. Unlike other patients in the sample, Gail had never experienced love and had little hope of attaining it. A second difference concerned Gail's high level of achievement. Patients with BPD, as in other categories of psychiatric illness, may suicide when they have great expectations that cannot be met.

Gail's early history is that of a temperamentally abnormal child. She might conceivably have benefited from being raised by parents with a greater capacity for empathy and support. The family was entirely successful in raising an easy child (Gail's older brother)—but not this very difficult one. The parents, probably realizing that they were not helpful, encouraged Gail's attempts to separate and to find another life far away from them. It is not clear whether Gail experienced their position as helpful. Unfortunately, she lacked the skills to build social networks and obtain the support she needed to achieve lasting independence.

With her anxious attachment, Gail became unusually dependent on therapists. Some patients with BPD center their lives completely on treatment, creating a safe haven until they feel ready to find another relationship. This process works best when the patient elicits a protective and caring response from the therapist. In Gail's case, she succeeded only in repeating her previous quarrels with her parents, and her outrageous behavior led her therapists to reject her. The breach with her last psychiatrist seems to have been a last straw leading to her completed suicide.

Case 16

Susan had seen a psychiatrist for the first time at age 20 years after dropping out of school, after which she was unemployed, could not leave home, and felt depressed. Her first hospital admission occurred after an overdose when she was 26 years old, but she remembered having wanted to die as long as she can remember. Susan was to remain in treatment for many years to come, and she made three serious suicide attempts that required intensive care.

Like many patients with BPD, Susan received a variety of diagnoses over the years, such as recurrent unipolar depression, schizotypal personality, and "pseudo-neurotic schizophrenia." What most contradicted the concept of a primary Axis I diagnosis was the fact that her illness showed no periods of remission. She had been treated over the years with a variety of tricylics and selective serotonin reuptake inhibitors, with little effect except for short-term improvement immediately following the change of medication.

Susan had severe problems, was difficult to treat, and also had bad luck with her therapists. Her first psychiatrist, who had bipolar illness, committed suicide after seeing her for a year. Her next two therapists discontinued treatment because of a lack of progress. Her fourth psychiatrist, whom she saw for 15 years, also had bipolar illness. After his death, for the last 10 years of her life, Susan attended the hospital clinic as an outpatient, seeing several different therapists.

Susan came from a difficult family. Both of her parents, as well as all three of her siblings, had received psychiatric treatment for depression, and both her father and brother had been admitted to hospitals. In her late 20s,

Susan married a businessman. He also appeared to suffer from depressive episodes and was treated with antidepressants. Their relationship was chronically troubled, and their sexual life was particularly unsatisfying. Susan's two sons had both been seen by a psychologist for learning difficulties, but they eventually completed school and moved out in their early 20s when they found jobs.

Susan had never held a job. Her life centered around home, although she had been doing volunteer work sporadically in recent years. She also had few friends. An additional stressor in the last years of her life was her declining health—she had been treated successfully for lung cancer but was discouraged by the experience.

The clinical notes prior to her death indicate that she was feeling increasingly hopeless, particularly after the departure of her children. The psychiatrist in the clinic referred her to the day hospital, which she accepted. However, while waiting to be admitted, she took a large quantity of clomipramine (which she had been hoarding) and was found dead by her husband on a morning when she had an appointment with her psychiatrist.

Comments

Susan was the oldest person (age 56) in our sample to commit suicide. Like many other patients with BPD, she felt she could not consider suicide as long as she had the responsibility for children. Susan had wished herself dead for most of her life. The departure of her boys left her with little—a husband to whom she was not close and no career to fall back on. Under these circumstances, ending her life became an option that she acted on.

Summary

These clinical narratives describe a very wide range of outcomes. The overall long-term outlook for BPD is reasonably good for an illness that is both severe and chronic. Although many patients have residual difficulties, clinicians can accept and feel pleased with a partial recovery.

7

Mechanisms of
Recovery

As Chapters 5 and 6 have shown, most patients with borderline personality disorder (BPD) eventually recover. Partial improvement seems to be the rule in Cluster B disorders, even in patients with antisocial personality disorder (ASPD). But what is the mechanism? Why can it take decades for improvement to set in?

This chapter suggests four general principles to explain the long-term outcome for patients with Cluster B personality disorders. The first is biological maturation. Over time, the natural course of impulsive traits is a decline in intensity, accompanied by increased behavioral control. The second is learning. However slowly they change, maladaptive behaviors respond to reinforcements. The third involves the avoidance of stressful situations such as intense intimate relationships. The fourth concerns developing adequate social supports and attaining a comfortable identity.

Biological Maturation

Impulsivity can be adaptive or maladaptive, depending on the circumstances. Life has always been full of danger. This was particularly true during the Paleolithic Era, when the human species evolved. Rapid responses to environmental challenges would have helped in situations such as hunting, escape from predators, challenges from competitors, or protection of young children. Yet, as with any trait, the value of a rapid response depends on context. There are times when a slow response, associated with anxiety and withdrawal, is more adaptive, because an individual with these traits is less likely to be exposed to acute danger. Thus, different behavioral patterns can be adaptive under different environmental conditions.

For this reason, evolution favors a range of characteristics that vary within a population. Personality traits follow this rule: They differ widely between individuals, and their effects on adaptation are context dependent.

Let us consider an example. In the New York Longitudinal Study, Chess and Thomas (1984) described the most common temperamental pattern in infants as "easy"—that is, a child who is responsive, not easily irritable, and readily comforted. In contrast, a minority of children, who are more irritable, were described as "difficult." There was also a third group, described as "slow to warm up." When times are good, it is better for both mother and child if the infant has an easy temperament. However, when times are not good, as deVries (1994) showed in African populations subject to times of famine, the "difficult" child, who makes more demands on the mother, is more likely to be fed and therefore to survive.

These variations developed many thousands of years ago, in an "environment of evolutionary adaptiveness" (Tooby and Cosmides 1992), but the same traits may not be useful in modern life. We no longer live as hunter-gatherers, pastoralists, or agriculturalists. In the contemporary world, attaining gainful employment requires very different skills, such as typing information into a computer. Even when a mild degree of impulsivity is useful (as it might be for soldiers or stock traders), overly rapid responses carry a measurable risk.

Evolution has shaped us to be more impulsive in youth than we are later in life. Youth is characterized by greater energy and less patience. This pattern actually makes practical sense. Hunter-gatherers have a high death rate as children, but those who reach maturity can achieve a long life span (Lee 1978). People lose physical strength with time but gain in experience, making it likely that they will be useful to the younger generation, particularly their relatives.

Most people note these changes in their own lives. We are much less impulsive at 40 than we were at 20. Clinicians observe parallel changes in their patients. If everyone becomes less impulsive with time, we should not be surprised to see less alcoholism, less bulimia, and less antisocial and borderline pathology in older people. By middle age, substance abusers are less likely to abuse substances, and criminals less likely to commit crimes. With time, patients with ASPD become less predatory and patients with BPD become less suicidal.

We do not know the precise mechanisms associated with these changes. Some may be biological, others psychological or social. Let us look at three possible biological mechanisms: changes in central serotonergic activity, increased myelinization, and rewiring of brain circuitry.

Changes in brain serotonin activity can lead to reductions in impulsive traits over time. Links between impulsivity and reduced serotonergic activity are the strongest and most consistent association between any personality trait and any specific neurotransmitter (Mann 1998). Moreover, it is known that serotonin activity increases with age (Leventhal 1996). It would therefore be interesting to study patients whose impulsive disorders burn out to determine whether standard measures of serotonin activity (e.g., challenge tests or positron emission tomography scans) demonstrate changes when repeated over a period of years. It is also possible that changes in other neurotransmitter systems, interacting with serotonergic pathways, play a role in reducing impulsive behaviors.

A second mechanism might involve neuroanatomical development. Vaillant (1977) hypothesized that reductions in impulsivity over time might be associated with completion of brain myelinization, which occurs in middle age. At present, there are few data supporting a link between this process and behavioral maturation.

Finally, the brain may be rewired over time. It has been found (Quartz and Sejnowski 1997) that neural connections are far from fixed and that new ones are shaped by events throughout the life span.

Yet none of these mechanisms explains why other mental disorders, ranging from schizophrenia to panic attacks, also become less common in early or late middle age (see Chapter 1). There must be other changes in brain function over time, but our present knowledge of neurobiology is insufficient to understand them.

Social Learning

Impulsivity interferes with learning. In spite of past experience, the man who has alcoholism convinces himself that he can handle one more drink. Even after a purge, the woman who has bulimia convinces herself that she can stay thin by dieting. The man with a gambling addiction returns to the table convinced that with just one more try, he will have a big win.

Yet however slow they are to learn, people with impulsive patterns of behavior can eventually get the point. The process by which people are shaped by direct reinforcements or influenced by seeing behaviors modeled by important people in their lives is called *social learning* (Bandura 1977). These mechanisms drive changes in behavior in children, and social learning continues throughout the life cycle.

Learning probably explains some of the changes observed by Black's group in their cohort of patients with ASPD. With age, these men had less energy to continue manipulating others. It is also possible that they learned to give up behaviors that consistently led to negative consequences. Thus, patients with ASPD can eventually learn how to stay on the right side of the law, and some may even learn how to keep a job or maintain a relationship.

In the same way, learning can account for improved functioning in BPD. With time, these patients may gradually learn to find ways to modulate their emotions, to avoid acting out impulsively, and to choose better partners for close relationships.

Similarly, learning can lead to a decreasing intensity of narcissistic traits. Life has a way of deflating most people's grandiosity. (Only those rare individuals with an unbroken pattern of success will be exceptions.) People with narcissistic personality disorder (NPD) may eventually learn that expecting perfection in life leads to disaster, particularly in intimate relationships. Patients with NPD often deal with conflict by changing partners. With time, however, patients with NPD may learn to become more tolerant and less demanding, accepting both their own achievements and the qualities of other people as "good enough."

Avoidance of Conflictual Intimacy

Patients with BPD have tumultuous and unstable relationships. To avoid making the same mistakes time after time, they must either slow down, exert better judgment, or simply avoid intimacy they cannot handle. By doing so, they can break the cyclic patterns that reinforce impulsivity and affective instability.

After interviewing 100 patients with BPD in our 15-year follow-up study, my colleague, Ron Brown, had the impression that many had improved functioning by avoiding conflicts brought on by intimacy. These people learned over time to be cautious about becoming attached too quickly, and they no longer put themselves in situations where this was likely to happen. By staying out of contexts that gave them particular trouble, patients with BPD were making a bargain. On the one hand, they restricted their options and experienced some degree of social isolation. On the other hand, by eliminating the triggers that brought on symptoms, they reached a point at which they no longer met criteria for BPD.

My own conclusions from conducting the interviews in the 27-year follow-up study were very similar. Moreover, many clinicians with long experience in monitoring patients with BPD, as well as colleagues who have conducted research on the long-term outcome for BPD, have expressed agreement, although we lack precise measures to prove this hypothesis correct.

I presented several clinical examples of this mechanism in Chapter 6. Although many subjects in our study felt lonely, they were relieved to be free of the tumult and chaos of their youth. In some cases, they were able to find other types of social bonds to replace intimacy. Many spoke of important friends, with whom they did not have to live. Others described strong relationships with pets. Still others reported a sense of belonging through joining a church or other community organizations.

Intimacy is dangerous for patients with BPD. As shown by Stone's (1990) study and by ours, marriage and parenthood are less common than in the general population. We also know from research on those who do have children (Feldman et al. 1995; Weiss et al. 1996) that parenting can be a very difficult task. Of course, some succeed. I provided an example in Chapter 6 of a patient ("Ellen") whose commitment to her children helped her overcome a severely traumatic childhood. On the other hand, I have seen some patients enter into "borderline relationships" with their children, demonstrating needy and clinging behaviors that interfere with the child's individuation and growth. We know that many patients with BPD have been raised by parents who have either BPD or other impulsive spectrum disorders (Links et al. 1988).

In summary, a significant minority of patients with BPD are able to achieve, and to benefit from, intimate relationships. However, a larger number choose to reject these options and seek out a niche in which their interpersonal deficits are not crippling.

Development of Social Support and Attainment of Identity

Recovery from Cluster B personality disorders requires a social support system. Yet in modern societies, support does not come automatically; it has to be sought out.

Impulsivity is a trait with high social sensitivity. Impulsive patients lack an inner sense of identity and coherence and therefore need more external structure. As discussed in Chapter 1, traditional cultures provide more structure than do modern societies, offering protection and buffering that limit the expression of impulsive behaviors. These structures make it easier to achieve employment as well as intimacy. Modern societies have a relative lack of structure and predictability, so that individuals need to create their own social roles as well as find their own partners. It should therefore not be surprising that patients presenting with ASPD and BPD have increased in prevalence in recent decades (Millon 1993; Paris 1996).

Lykken (1995) emphasized how sensitive antisocial traits are to vagaries in the socialization process. Linehan (1993) suggested that increases in the prevalence of BPD reflects decreases in social support for those who are emotionally vulnerable. Similarly, Kohut (1977) speculated that narcissistic pathology becomes more common as family and social structures become less effective in providing a sense of self.

Long-term outcome for these disorders should also be dependent on the availability of social supports. Traditionally, many of these supports were provided in the context of settled societies and organized religion. Modernity and the rise of individualistic values has limited attachment to community organizations (Millon 1993). Yet even today, those who can "find a home" in religion are protected from developing patterns of impulsive behaviors. On the basis of their long experience with men with ASPD admitted to a psychiatric hospital, Yochelson and Samenow (1976) came to the conclusion that religious conversion was almost the only way to achieve a stable recovery from ASPD. (I return to this issue in Chapter 8.)

In a semilegendary encounter, Carl Gustav Jung told a man (later known only as Bill) that he would recover from substance abuse only if he found his way back to God. Bill was a stockbroker who, along with a physician who had alcoholism, founded Alcoholics Anonymous (AA), which used many of the elements of traditional religion (in an overtly Protestant context) to build a powerful social movement. AA is still the most effective way of combating alcoholism (Vaillant 1995), and its methods have been copied by Narcotics Anonymous, Gamblers Anonymous, and Overeaters Anonymous, as well as by the entire support group movement.

The secret of AA is that it provides high levels of support (weekly meetings and 24-hour availability of a sponsor). It also has an ethos that requires members to surrender individualistic illusions—that is, to accept that the lure of the bottle is stronger than they are and to consign their future to a "higher power." Finally, substance abusers are provided with structure and a sense of responsibility for the consequences of behavior. As drug counselors know from long experience, these clients need "tough love," not sympathy.

In BPD, one of the reasons why patients may not do well in "classical" open-ended therapy is that they do not tolerate an unstructured treatment. Stern (1938), the first writer to describe patients with BPD, identified their failure to respond to psychoanalysis. Stern noted great difficulty tolerating the expectation to lie on a couch and to free associate. In contrast, the success of Linehan (1993) in keeping most patients in treatment could well be attributable to her highly structured approach. Any successful treatment of impulsive disorders must incorporate these basic elements of structure and support.

Some patients with BPD find and maintain social supports, even without formal treatment. Chapter 6 provided several examples of this mechanism. About half of our patients with BPD were living in stable relationships, whereas another half had not achieved intimacy. Yet we saw two pathways to gaining stable social supports: through an intimate relationship and/or a family and through friendship and community organizations. As patients' impulsivity declined, and as they learned to manage relationships better, they were able to sustain bonds, whether intimate or nonintimate— sometimes after years of bouncing from one unstable situation to another.

Social support also helps people to become comfortable with who they are (i.e., forming an identity), even when they are notably different from others. Identity problems are a basic feature of BPD; therefore, finding a purpose in life and feeling comfortable with oneself should be basic to recovery.

Sexual orientation is an interesting example of this process. Patients with BPD are somewhat more likely than the general population to be homosexual or bisexual. We observed that 10% of men with BPD had a stable homosexual orientation (Paris et al. 1995), a finding confirmed by two other groups (Dulit et al. 1993; Zubenko et al. 1987). In females with BPD (Paris et al. 1994a), the rate of homosexual preference was 4%. In the community, stable homosexual preference ranges around 2% for males and 1% for females (Michaels 1996). We also observed many examples of bisexuality: The rate for any homosexual contact among the men was 16% and 18% among the women. In the community, the frequency of homosexual contact in the course of a lifetime is 7% for males and 3% for females (Michaels 1996). Although the community prevalence of BPD and other Cluster B disorders in this population is unknown, these traits could account, at least in part, for the high prevalence of suicide attempts in the homosexual community (Herrell et al. 1999).

Some of the patients in our follow-up cohort who were homosexual had remarkable improvement in functioning when they came out—that is, when they firmly established and felt comfortable with an orientation. Social attitudes about these issues have changed dramatically since the time when these patients were first seen. Prior to 1970, homosexuality was considered to be a mental disorder, and the psychiatric literature contained many discussions concerning the best way to treat this "illness." As a result, many suffered unnecessarily.

In Chapter 6 I described "Tom," a young man with all the typical symptoms of BPD who made a complete and sustained recovery when he moved to another large city and established a lifestyle supported by the gay community. In our 27-year follow-up study, 6 of the 64 subjects given a follow-up interview were homosexual in orientation (4 women and 2 men), for a rate of 9%. At this point in their lives, none reported further conflict about their sexuality.

Conclusions

The mechanisms of recovery in Cluster B personality disorders are multiple. As patients grow older, they become less impulsive. Most learn either to manage intimacy or to find a way to avoid it. Social supports and the resolution of identity problems also lead to remission.

Essentially, recovery for these patients is a compromise that works. Unfortunately, this process may not be effective for those with Cluster A and Cluster C disorders, who can become locked into painful isolation.

8

Course, Prevention, and Management

This chapter addresses some practical implications of the research reviewed in this book. I address here a wide range of questions: 1) What is the relevance of identifying childhood precursors, and can we prevent personality disorders from developing? 2) Is there good evidence for the effectiveness of psychotherapy in personality disorders? 3) In light of the chronicity of personality disorders, is long-term treatment required? 4) How useful are pharmacological interventions? 5) What other methods are helpful for patients with personality disorders? 6) Does treatment influence long-term outcome?

Can Personality Disorders Be Prevented?

In the 1960s, a great surge of optimism pervaded the mental health professions. We thought we knew the most important causes of mental disorders: poor parenting and social disadvantage. To prevent psychopathology, community psychiatrists and other professionals proposed programs to teach parents how to manage children and to improve socioeconomic conditions for the underclass. Why did this early stage of community psychiatry crash and burn? In part, because its aims were grandiose. Our view of the causes of disorders was also wrong. Family and social dysfunction are associated risk factors that carry an increased risk for psychopathology. By themselves, however, they do not cause mental illness. Instead, they make it more likely for vulnerable individuals to cross the boundary to overt disorders. The other problem with the community psychiatry of the past is that its programs, however well-meaning, lacked a firm base in evidence. Today, we take it for granted that the value of new forms of treatment must be proven

111

through empirical research. The same expectation should apply to preventive interventions, however plausible they seem.

Clinicians working with children have always had a strong interest in prevention. Child psychiatrists and developmental psychologists have learned that children with conduct disorder are at high risk for developing substance abuse and antisocial behavior as adults. But does this information allow us to prevent such outcomes?

To answer this question, we need to know whether early treatment makes a difference. In the short term, interventions with children who have conduct disorder (e.g., Vitaro and Tremblay 1994) have yielded encouraging results. However, many patients drop out of these programs, and improvements are not often maintained in the long term (Kazdin 2001). Given the chronicity of conduct symptoms, we must carry out follow-up studies to see if interventions during childhood can prevent adult sequelae. The problem is even more complex for disorders for which childhood precursors have not been identified. By and large, we do not know enough about the causes of mental illnesses to develop rational plans for preventing them.

At this point, I can only outline an approach that we might take once the data are in. The central issue is to define populations at risk. In the past, preventive programs (such as health education and community activities) have been offered to entire populations of children, most of whom have no significant psychopathology. This approach might be described as "preaching to the converted."

Prevention requires a *targeted* approach. It could be cost-effective to identify children who are most likely to develop disorders and to target our interventions to reach that population. We already know enough to identify groups that are high risk because of psychosocial adversities such as neglect and child abuse. In the future, we may also be able to use biological research to identify vulnerable populations. In the future, it may become routine to "read" every child's genome. Because personality traits are associated with genetic profiles, problematic characteristics such as impulsivity might be identified very early in life. Personality disorders emerge from gene–environment interactions, so we would ideally wish to target children who are at risk on both counts. Thus far, the most impressive research concerning prevention has come from a study by Olds et al. (1998). In a randomized, controlled trial with a 15-year follow-up period, it was found that regular nurse home visits to mothers, lasting from the time of birth to the child's second birthday, had a significant effect in reducing antisocial behavior and substance use in the children when they reached adolescence. This study used a highly targeted approach, actively recruiting young unmarried mothers, who formed the majority of the sample.

The findings of the study by Olds et al. need replication, and there was no formal follow-up evaluation of how the intervention affected the sample over the intervening 13 years. Nonetheless, home visits may have gotten these high-risk mothers off to a better start than otherwise would have been the case. It is also possible that the mothers who agreed to enter this study were more receptive than those we see in clinical situations. We do not know whether similar results could have been obtained in highly dysfunctional families or in children with abnormal temperament.

The coming decades could bring a new type of preventive psychiatry. To break the cycles that can spiral into personality disorders, we must identify precursors, target traits, and develop more effective ways of modifying them. We will need new ways of controlling impulsivity, requiring a combination of pharmacological and psychosocial interventions. We will also need to identify internalizing symptoms at an earlier stage and to find new ways of relieving distress in these children. We are decades away from being able to modify temperament, either through pharmacotherapy or gene therapy. At this point, therefore, our efforts at prevention must focus on the environment, but some aspects of risk are not likely to change. Socioeconomic improvements will not be enough. Many of those at greatest risk are locked into pathogenic environments. The breakdown of community institutions and of the family is unlikely to be reversed. Preventing disorders, even if it turns out to be possible, will be expensive.

Research on Psychotherapy for Personality Disorders

Is treatment or time more important in determining the outcome for patients with personality disorders? These are chronic conditions that wax and wane over the short term and may remit over the long term. How can we distinguish naturalistic improvement from true therapeutic effects? The ideal study would be a randomized, controlled trial with a large group of patients, with therapy lasting several years, comparing those treated with a defined method of psychotherapy with another group receiving little or no treatment. Such a project would be very expensive, and it might not even be ethical. The most practical research strategy up to now has depended on a more practical approach, comparing the effects of a defined intervention with "treatment as usual" in the community, the method used by Linehan (1993) to study dialectical behavior therapy (DBT). Unfortunately, the empirical literature on the treatment of personality disorders is restricted to only a few of the categories listed on Axis II, and the largest body of research concerns patients with borderline personality disorder (BPD).

Nonetheless, I begin with a discussion of antisocial personality disorder (ASPD) and also briefly examine other Axis II categories.

Antisocial Personality Disorder

Patients with ASPD are famously resistant to therapy, failing to respond to virtually every form of intervention that has been tried (Gabbard and Coyne 1987; Yochelson and Samenow 1976). In spite of some enthusiasm in the 1960s for milieu therapy in closed settings, the results remain very disappointing (see review in Black 1999). One problem is that patients are not well motivated for treatment. As several observers (Black 1999; Cleckley 1964; Harpur et al. 1994) have noted, patients with ASPD tend to present in a tight spot, hoping to manipulate the care system to escape responsibility for their actions. After many years of working with this population, Cleckley (1964) concluded he had little to offer them. In recent decades, however, a few devoted clinicians, particularly in forensic settings (e.g., Dolan and Coid 1993), have applied their skills treating patients with ASPD. Even so, we lack convincing clinical trials showing that any method of therapy is consistently effective over time. The follow-up study by Black et al. (1995) presented in Chapter 5 suggests that most patients retain severe deficits throughout their lives.

There can be exceptions to the rule. The experience of Yochelson and Samenow (1976), who worked at St. Elizabeth's Hospital in Washington, D.C. in the 1960s, is instructive. This was an unusual period in the District of Columbia, in that the "Durham rule" (a broadened insanity defense based on a case involving a defendant named Durham) was used to reduce criminal responsibility for actions resulting from almost any mental condition. Even a personality disorder was considered to be a mitigating factor by the courts in this jurisdiction, and a large number of patients with ASPD were admitted to the psychiatric hospital for treatment and rehabilitation.

Yochelson, a retired psychoanalyst, was recruited to run the program; Samenow, a clinical psychologist, joined him later. In their book, they described their attempts to treat patients with ASPD with psychotherapy. All of their efforts led to total failure. (Not too many books have been written elaborating such a theme!) It also became clear that many patients had been apprehended for only a very small percentage of their crimes and that few felt any remorse for their actions. Although the therapists observed that patients with ASPD can sometimes become suicidal if placed in solitary confinement (or some other setting from which they cannot escape), that state of mind does not last for long. Yochelson and Samenow deserve credit for pointing out that their own methods, as well as those of others in the field, were ineffective. Neither the work of Maxwell Jones (1953) with milieu therapy in England nor that of the Patuxent Institute in Maryland (Court-less 1997) produced lasting results. Patients simply tolerated the therapeutic milieu until they could be released, whereupon they resumed their previous activities. Yet Yochelson and Samenow did have a few patients whose disorder remitted. This happened when they succeeding in making patients feel *guilty* about their actions. This "superego transplant" resembled the methods that religious movements have traditionally used to convert the most deviant members of society.

One of my students, presented with this story, remarked that Yochelson and Samenow had rediscovered the Salvation Army! In a similar historical example, Malcolm Little, an antisocial young man with a long criminal record, converted to Islam and became Malcolm X, a highly effective political leader (Barr 1994). After an early trajectory that followed the classical paradigm for ASPD, Malcolm became a different person. Ironically, he was assassinated when he refused to become involved in crimes perpetrated by the movement he had joined.

As Robins (1966) emphasized, not all people with ASPD are hard-core criminals. Many are people who live on the margins of society and self-medicate dysphoria with street drugs. In a substance abuse clinic population, Woody et al. (1985) found that patients with ASPD who also meet criteria for a clinical diagnosis of depression (and who therefore have some capacity for guilt) can be helped in outpatient therapy. Nonetheless, the overall picture for patients with ASPD remains dismal. For clinicians who are not forensic specialists, making this diagnosis is mainly valuable to the extent that it provides a reason to avoid accepting patients into therapy. The abnormal traits in ASPD, when reinforced by psychosocial factors, are difficult to reverse. However maladaptive in the long run, manipulativeness will have yielded intermittent positive reinforcements. Even though the worst aspects burn out by middle age, recovered patients with ASPD have failed to undergo crucial periods of social learning, normally occurring in adolescence and young adulthood. These experiences help individuals develop skills in attaining stable employment and establishing meaningful intimate relationships. Taken together, these abnormal traits and lack of skills development leave the patients with a deficit that makes them continue antisocial behaviors, albeit at a lower level of intensity. For these reasons, ASPD remains difficult to treat, either at diagnosable levels in youth or at subdiagnostic levels in later life.

In the future, we will need different forms of therapy to manage ASPD. Some could be psychopharmacological, addressing the biology of the traits underlying the disorder (Masters and McGuire 1994). Another possibility could involve a cognitive-behavioral therapy specifically designed for psychopathy (Beck and Freeman 1990). Taken together, these abnormal traits and lack of skills development leave the patient with a deficit that makes them continue antisocial behaviors, albeit at a lower level of intensity. The method might well be similar to the techniques that Linehan (1993) developed to treat BPD. However, in a society that protects the individual's civil liberty to refuse treatment, patients with ASPD might well refuse effective therapeutic modalities, even if we had them. In spite of the recent decline in crime rates in the United States, we do not have any evidence that ASPD is becoming less common. Given the continuing role of social factors in the disorder, its prevalence will probably remain high (Robins and Regier 1991). At this point, naturalistic improvement may be the best we can hope for.

Borderline Personality Disorder

Patients with BPD richly deserve their reputation among clinicians for being troublesome and resistant to treatment. Yet the outlook for BPD is much more favorable than for ASPD. Research shows that patients with BPD often fail to respond to standard forms of psychotherapy. Studies of open-ended treatment (Gunderson et al. 1989; Skodol et al. 1983) demonstrate that when patients with BPD are offered long-term therapy, two-thirds drop out within a few months. This suggests that patients with BPD have difficulty tolerating unstructured treatment.

Perhaps this type of therapy should be restricted to the most treatable patients, those with higher levels of functioning (Paris 1994). Stevenson and Meares (1992) obtained much lower dropout rates (16%) in a subpopulation preselected as suitable for long-term dynamic therapy. Highly structured methods of treatment can lower the rate even further. In Linehan's (1993) controlled clinical trial of DBT, the frequency of dropouts fell below 10%.

Published reports describing the effectiveness of "classical" psychodynamic approaches to BPD (e.g., Adler 1985; Chessick 1985) have generally been based on case examples. These claims must be confirmed by clinical trials. Moreover, methods effective for patients in private practice may not be generalizable to the larger population with BPD in clinics. Research on the treatment of personality disorders at the Menninger Clinic (Wallerstein 1986), which probably included many patients with BPD, provided a systematic, albeit uncontrolled, follow-up evaluation of a treated sample. Ego strength prior to therapy (Kernberg et al. 1972) as well as the quality of the therapeutic alliance during treatment (Horwitz 1974) were the best predictors of a good outcome. However, the Menninger study had many limitations: It monitored only 42 subjects, lacked a control group, and provided no data on diagnosis.

The most important study of long-term psychoanalytic psychotherapy in BPD was conducted in Sydney, Australia, by Stevenson and Meares (1992). These researchers reported clear-cut improvement in a cohort of BPD patients after 2 years of therapy. The method was based on a self-psychology model, and followed standard psychodynamic principles. The original study had no control group, but Meares et al. (1999) later compared their results with outcome among a group of untreated control subjects left on a waiting list. Although this was not truly a controlled trial, after 1 year 30% of the treated group, and none of the control subjects, lost their diagnosis of BPD. These results show that therapy is better than no therapy. However, the generalizability of these findings to clinical practice was limited by the absence of randomization and by failure to compare the cohort in therapy with a group receiving treatment as usual.

Other data suggesting that well-structured psychodynamic therapy can yield good results have come from studies by Sabo et al. (1995) and Najavits and Gunderson (1995). These reports showed that cohorts of patients with BPD in open-ended dynamic therapy show significant declines in self-harm within a year. However, because neither of these studies used a comparison group, we cannot know whether improvements were specific to the treatment method or whether they might have occurred without treatment.

The only randomized controlled trial of psychodynamic treatment has been conducted by Bateman and Fonagy (1999) in a day treatment unit that treated patients with individual and group therapy for up to 18 months. This report found clear-cut improvement in BPD, and the results were stable at 1-year follow-up evaluation (Bateman and Fonagy 2001). Although these findings are very encouraging, it is not clear whether positive results were due to the structure of day treatment or to the psychotherapy. The authors are presently carrying out a trial of outpatient treatment that may help to clarify this question.

Few studies of outpatient therapy for personality disorders have used control groups, but Linehan's work is a striking exception (Linehan et al. 1991). She showed DBT to be clearly superior to "treatment as usual" (outpatient therapy in the community). After a year of treatment, those undergoing DBT were less likely to make suicide gestures and spent less time in hospitals. However, at 2-year follow-up evaluation, the groups were more similar. On one outcome measure (frequency of parasuicide), there was no difference at 2 years, though the group treated with DBT continued to have a higher functional level. Moreover, most patients treated with DBT stayed in therapy for the full year, although they did receive free treatment, whereas the cohort in treatment as usual did not. These results were later replicated in a group of substance-abusing patients with BPD (Koerner and Linehan 2002).

We need replication studies of DBT in larger samples, and in settings not linked to Linehan's team. At present the original results have been replicated in small samples of patients from two other centers (Koons et al. 2001; Sanderson et al. 2002) as well as a larger replication from the Netherlands (Verheul et al. 2003). It also remains possible that selection biases could have affected the generalizability of Linehan's results. Although Linehan has emphasized that her team took on some of the most difficult patients in the community, not every patient with BPD will follow through with DBT; it is not clear how the research team sifted the patients before accepting them into the project. However encouraging the results of existing trials of treatment for BPD, we do not know whether they are generalizable to the larger clinical population (Scheel 2000). Many patients with BPD will not continue with therapy in any consistent way. Results from patients preselected for long-term therapy cannot be generalized to everyone. In a commentary on the study by Meares et al. (1999), Allen (1999) wondered whether the enthusiasm and support associated with research studies might also partially account for a positive outcome. Similar questions could be raised about the results of the Linehan study.

Currently, DBT is the best-documented treatment for BPD. However, because comparative trials have not been conducted, we do not know whether it is superior to psychodynamic therapy. It is premature to assume that there is one best form of psychotherapy for patients with BPD. I have often heard Linehan argue that because her method has proven its efficacy, clinicians suggesting the use of other approaches need to carry out parallel research to support their methods. In practice, however, it is hard to be sure whether the results of DBT are better, or better documented.

Clearly, more research is needed about the usefulness of psychological treatment for patients with BPD. On the positive side, these findings show that psychotherapy *can* be effective in BPD. These results contradict the pessimism that many clinicians associate with a diagnosis of BPD.

However, there are practical problems in prescribing psychotherapy for BPD. Some patients cannot readily be engaged in treatment. Others cannot pay for it. Linehan's trials of DBT were supported by a large grant from the National Institute of Mental Health. In the 10 years since her results were published, many therapists have trained in her method, and a list is available on the Internet. However, the treatment is not free. The same consideration applies to psychodynamic therapy, whose scope has long been limited by its expense.

Many patients with BPD receive welfare subsidies, and those who are working are usually far from wealthy. In the United States, managed care has pulled the rug out from beneath insured long-term psychotherapy (even if some therapists in public clinics still offer open-ended treatment).

In Europe, government insurance does not generally cover extensive psychotherapy. In Canada, where I work, all forms of psychotherapy of whatever length are paid for by provincial health insurance. However, this insurance covers only psychiatrists, only a few of whom have large psychotherapy practices. Most patients with BPD still cannot find therapists who provide open-ended therapy unless they (the patients) can pay.

The American Psychiatric Association Guidelines for the Treatment of Borderline Personality Disorder

The American Psychiatric Association (APA) has published the "Practice Guideline for the Treatment of Borderline Personality Disorder" (American Psychiatric Association 2001). In 2002, I edited a section in the *Journal of Personality Disorders* containing responses from several experts about these guidelines. I summarize the comments here.

British psychiatrist Peter Tyrer (2002) pointed out that we need to apply standard criteria used in other practice guidelines (Sackett et al. 1997), with five levels of evidence ranked hierarchically: 1) systematic review of randomized controlled trials with meta-analyses, 2) single randomized controlled trials, 3) quasi-randomized studies; 4) nonexperimental descriptive studies, and 5) expert opinion. Tyrer noted that none of the recommendations in the APA report was based on level 1 data and that the few randomized controlled trials that do exist have not been replicated.

Other commentators in the journal issue came to similar conclusions. McGlashan (2002) considered the limited data on psychotherapy for BPD to be inconclusive. Sanderson et al. (2002), representing the DBT community, strongly criticized the report for applying a lower standard to dynamic therapy and a higher one to cognitive therapy.

The senior author of the APA report (Oldham 2002) emphasized that the very publication of such a document is a milestone that recognizes a certain level of progress in personality disorder research. Perhaps conclusions should be held in abeyance until more data are forthcoming. However, given the available evidence, Peter Tyrer (2002) was right to remark, rather wittily, that the guidelines are "a bridge too far."

I agree with the critics that an APA practice guideline should have been more cautious in its conclusions. (Having seen previous versions of this document as a consultant, I credit John Oldham for reducing the large amount of clinical opinion that afflicted earlier drafts.) However, one cannot practice psychiatry in full accordance with evidence-based standards. We need much more research on these issues. As a clinician, I tend to agree with the broad conclusions of the guideline: There is sufficient evidence to conclude that psychotherapy should be offered to patients with BPD when it is available. Unless there is a clear contraindication, we have enough evidence supporting psychological interventions to make them worth a try.

We do not have evidence that the theoretical basis of therapy makes a crucial difference in outcome. For patients with BPD, it may be most important to offer treatment that is consistent and well-structured. Such patients seem to need a strong dose of the common or "nonspecific" elements of psychotherapy. These factors support a strong therapeutic alliance and a positive relationship, which are the most effective ingredients in psychotherapy (see reviews in Bergin and Garfield 1994). These elements may be of even greater importance for patients with BPD who lack outside supports.

One of the great strengths of DBT is that it specifies the nonspecific factors in treatment, with the goal of maximizing them. However, all good clinicians learn to practice in accordance with these principles. Whatever their background and training, therapists who succeed with patients with BPD must be positive, practical, and empathic.

Other Personality Disorders

Although there is controversy about the level of evidence needed to reach conclusions about psychotherapy for BPD, the situation is much worse for other categories of personality disorder. Other than trials of social skills training for patients with avoidant personality disorder (e.g., Alden 1989), we have very little go to on.

There has been some research examining the effectiveness of psychotherapy in mixed cohorts of patients with diagnoses falling into various categories of personality disorder. Monsen et al. (1995) found that many patients attain clinical improvement after 2 years of therapy, with most losing their initial diagnoses. However, the conclusions of that study were limited by the absence of a control group. Again, this makes it difficult to determine whether improvements after psychotherapy reflect naturalistic remission or true treatment effects.

In a study of patients with anxious cluster and histrionic personality disorders (Winston et al. 1994), the results were similar to those of the Sydney study of BPD—that is, significant improvement after 40 sessions of therapy, as compared with those left untreated on a waiting list. Efficacy would have been better established, however, if the results had been compared with those for a group receiving treatment as usual.

The overall effectiveness of psychotherapy for personality disorders has been examined using meta-analytic methods. One meta-analysis of treatment studies of patients with personality disorders (Perry et al. 1999) compared the results of therapy with rates of naturalistic recovery found in follow-up research. Perry et al. estimated that each year, 3.7% of patients naturally recover from impulsive personality disorders. On the basis of four studies that assessed diagnoses at the end of treatment, the authors concluded that therapy leads to a 25.8% remission rate per year and that improvement with therapy occurs at a much more rapid rate than would have occurred otherwise.

Although I agree with Perry's group that the evidence for psychotherapy in the personality disorders is encouraging, the conclusions in this article were overly optimistic. The first problem is that the data set depended on what was available in the literature, which is sparse. Second, the meta-analysis included a wide a range of diagnoses, with 5 studies of BPD and 10 of other categories of personality disorder. Third, most of the studies were either uncontrolled or partially controlled, raising questions as to whether improvement was related to treatment. Fourth, the meta-analysis combined studies using a wide variety of methods, including dynamic therapy (e.g., Høglend 1993; Monsen et al. 1995; Stevenson and Meares 1992), cognitive therapy (Linehan 1993), and short-term group therapy (Budman et al. 1996). Finally, in light of other data, the estimate by Perry et al. of 3.7% recovery per year for personality disorders is probably too low.

Changes in diagnostic status have to be measured against the natural instability of personality disorder diagnoses over time (McDavid and Pilkonis 1996). Vaglum et al. (1996) found that as many as 30% of patients with BPD no longer meet criteria at 2- to 5-year follow–up evaluation. The National Institute of Mental Health Collaborative Study of Personality Disorders (Grilo et al. 2000) also found that about one-third of patients with BPD fall below the level of DSM-IV (American Psychiatric Association 1994) criteria within 1–2 years. It is not clear whether these changes represent true recovery or the waxing and waning of a chronic illness in response to life events. In addition to diagnosis, we would need to know how well patients are functioning and whether they are likely to relapse when faced with new adversities.

In summary, research underlies the need to be cautious about drawing general conclusions on the overall effectiveness of treatment for personality disorders. This is a broad and heterogeneous group of patients, some of whom are treatable and some of whom are not. Moreover, existing research has to be replicated in larger and more representative samples. As a clinician, I have had the experience that therapy works quite well for *some* patients. These could be the same people who are most likely to enter and remain in research studies. Yet my clinical experience, as well as my studies of the long-term outcome of BPD, also tells me that therapies that work for some patients are *not* very effective for others. Therefore, the prescription of therapy should not be routine, but individualized.

Length of Psychotherapy in Light of Long-Term Outcome

I have often heard colleagues say that patients who have been dysfunctional for many years need an equally lengthy treatment. This assumption is most common among psychodynamic therapists but has also been endorsed by cognitive therapists interested in personality disorders. Both Linehan (1993) and Young (1999) state that the treatment of BPD requires several years and that the partial improvements they describe in their follow-up studies are only the first steps on the road to recovery.

A report by Høglend (1993) offered support for the idea that patients with personality disorders need more than the 10- to 20-session therapy frequently prescribed in clinics. In this cohort, patients with an Axis II diagnosis had improved function when the treatment lasted for 50 sessions. Similar findings emerged from a study of large populations undergoing treatment at psychological clinics in the United States (Kopta et al. 1994). A more disturbed subgroup labeled, without much diagnostic precision, as "borderline-psychotic," required more time to attain symptomatic improvement, whereas "characterological" symptoms, such as hostility, paranoid trends, or an inability to get close to other people all required longer therapy. Nonetheless, even when allowed to take more time, only 50% of these patients actually recovered after a year of therapy. Thus, although longer courses were more likely to be effective, patients did not always benefit from them.

Again, research does not support a blanket recommendation for open-ended therapy for patients with personality disorders. To do so would fail to distinguish between those who benefit most and those who benefit least. As every clinician knows, patients can be monitored for years on end without great effect. This is an expensive procedure, and therapy of this duration is usually an option only for those who can afford to pay.

Moreover, extended treatment does not appeal to all patients. Many are more comfortable with intermittent therapy (McGlashan 1993). The patients who stay in therapy for many years are not necessarily representative of the larger population with personality disorders. Some seek open-ended treatment because of a lack of social supports, so that therapy becomes a replacement for a community, providing a safe haven from a rejecting world.

At the end of his career, Freud (1937/1964) acknowledged that psychoanalysis, given its indefinite goals, has a tendency to become interminable. This problem was well documented in the Menninger study (Horwitz 1974; Wallerstein 1986). As one might expect in a naturalistic study, some patients were fully recovered, some were partially recovered, and some remained continuously symptomatic. However, a good number of the patients in the Menninger cohort became "lifers," in that they saw therapy as a necessity in their lives and had no expectation of *ever* terminating. Obviously, they could afford to pay for lifelong treatment.

Long-term therapy can sometimes become a "mission impossible," aiming to cure problems that can, at best, only be ameliorated. Some clinicians have been taught not to discharge patients until the treatment is "complete." When patients fail to improve, and if the therapist believes that relapse will follow discharge, supportive care can continue, even over a lifetime. One of my teachers used to see a patient with BPD who was well known in the building where I work. She spent many hours there, chatting with secretaries and receptionists. My teacher was a training analyst, and the patient was wealthy enough to pay for his services. He described the situation as follows: "The treatment will only end when one of us dies. The only question is who will go first." (The therapist went first, and the patient sought treatment elsewhere.)

The long-term outcome for BPD places its therapy in a different light. McGlashan (1993) published a set of treatment recommendations based on the findings of his 15-year follow-up study of patients with BPD. Given that these patients gradually recover but remain fragile, McGlashan saw intermittent therapy as the "default position." Specifically, he recommended that clinicians should allow patients to enter and leave therapy as they fall in and out of serious difficulty. Because it often takes time to establish an alliance with patients who have personality disorders, the longest period of treatment would be the first one, after which each subsequent period could be shorter.

McGlashan's approach has another advantage: It allows patients to discharge themselves without having to leave against advice. This leaves an open door for those who have trouble coping with ambivalence and dependency in the therapeutic relationship. In a survey of experienced psychotherapists treating patients with BPD, Waldinger and Gunderson (1984) found that many patients in open-ended treatment left against the wishes of the therapist, who wanted to continue for longer. One wonders if patients are more readily satisfied with partial results than their therapists.

Silver (1983), a researcher who has conducted a follow-up study of patients with BPD, came to similar conclusions about clinical care. He advised that patients need to complete "a piece of work" and attain a degree of closure, after which they can be encouraged to try things on their own for a while. Because this approach requires rapid access for reentry, it should not be undertaken by therapists who maintain rigid schedules.

My own views on the treatment of patients with BPD have been strongly influenced by my involvement in long-term outcome research. At our

27-year follow-up evaluation, only 28% of our subjects were still in treatment. Some, but not all, of these patients were highly symptomatic. Most of the rest were doing reasonably well without continuous therapy. Patients with BPD need to retain ready access to treatment, but this need not mean they have to attend weekly sessions indefinitely.

Another factor driving interminable therapy is the belief that patients do get better until they "work through" their unhappy childhood. Yet some aspects of the past can never be worked though—one just has to move on. Moreover, an atmosphere conducive to a reparenting experience inevitably encourages dependency, regression, and impasse. Finally, prescribing lifelong therapy communicates the wrong message. Instead of encouraging autonomy, we make patients feel they cannot do without us. Whose needs does that serve?

In my experience, patients can usually be weaned down to less frequent visits, as long as they know the therapist will be available in a crisis. Some will maintain contact by dropping by every so often; others simply by sending their ex-therapist a yearly greeting card. Still others may prefer not to be in touch unless they need a "retread."

Ideally, intermittent therapy should be carried out by the same clinician, who benefits from knowing the patient's problems in detail. In practice, this does not always happen. Patients or their therapists can relocate. Or patients with BPD who use splitting defenses may develop a pattern of rejecting one therapist and then seeking out another. Most of us who treat this population have been on the receiving end of these rejections, which sometimes leave us feeling wounded but can also leave us feeling relieved. Yet changing therapists need not always be a bad thing. Wolberg (1973) thought that patients have to go through many treatments before they attain the normal degree of ambivalence that allows most people to remain in a therapeutic relationship. Yet there is probably a simpler explanation—patients may improve over time, leaving the last therapist with all the credit! The following clinical example illustrates this scenario.

> Clara, a senior medical student, consulted me at the University Health Service. She had been overtly rejected by her previous therapist, Dr. W., who abruptly informed her she did not need any further treatment. However, Clara remained chronically suicidal, had intermittent psychotic episodes, and had been socially isolated since adolescence.
>
> Dr. W. was an experienced psychiatrist with a special interest in patients with personality disorders and had been one of my most esteemed teachers. He had been treating Clara for 3 years and was initially very giving with her, allowing her to call him at home several times a week and providing her with extra sessions for crises. In the course of treatment, Dr. W. prescribed almost every current antidepressant, neuroleptic, and benzodiazepine for Clara. He also hospitalized her whenever she was suicidal (which occurred

several times) and used his influence at the medical school to get her past various academic hurdles.

Clara idolized Dr. W. but was unable to stop being importunate. Gradually, he became more and more burned out by her demands. The last straw came when Dr. W. was himself hospitalized for a cholecystectomy. The last person Dr. W., groggy and in pain, wanted to see in his room was Clara, but Clara felt that she had to make sure her therapist was all right. After this incident, their relationship went rapidly downhill. Once Clara was discharged from his care, Dr. W. spent the rest of his career focusing on the pharmacological treatment of patients with schizophrenia and bipolar illness.

Dr. W. was Clara's fourth therapist. She had been in continuous treatment since midadolescence, spending about a year with a series of well-regarded psychiatrists, each of whom she found inadequate. Aware that I was now the fifth therapist, I aimed to set a few simple goals—prescribing minimal medication, avoiding hospitalization, and concentrating on getting Clara through the last year of medical school. Although she never became deeply attached to me, Clara tolerated my supportive approach, and I carried her to graduation and through a rotating internship.

When Clara moved to another city to undertake a residency in family practice, she arranged to see a colleague known for his clinical interest in patients with BPD. At this point, my own view of her future prospects was cautious. If she was able to practice her profession, I thought, work might at least provide a buffer against chronic loneliness. Because she had never had an intimate relationship, I thought it unlikely she would ever have one.

Some years later, I ran into Clara's sixth therapist. When I asked him how she was doing, his answer surprised me. Clara was practicing medicine and was also married and had three children. Her only residual symptom involved hypochondriacal preoccupations that led her to seek the advice of other physicians. When I asked my colleague how he had achieved so much, he described have taken a very firm line on boundaries and getting Clara focused on problem-solving.

Several possibilities come to mind about this outcome. The last therapist may have been more skilled than any of his predecessors. Clara may have reached a point when she could benefit from therapy without behaving in ways that undermined her treatment. Finally, Clara's borderline pathology may simply have burned out early.

Psychopharmacology in Cluster B Personality Disorders

Outcome research also provides a frame for assessing the usefulness of psychopharmacology in patients with personality disorders. The issue is much the same as it was for psychotherapy: How can we evaluate the efficacy of treatment in patients who are chronically ill and whose disorder has a waxing and waning course? In short, how can we be sure that these interventions are truly effective?

Almost all of the research in psychopharmacology has focused on BPD, and it must be approached cautiously. Few of these studies were randomized controlled trials. Most have used small samples, probably because it is not easy to recruit patients with BPD for clinical research.

Table 8–1 summarizes the findings of published randomized placebo-controlled trials for BPD. A variety of agents were used; effects on mood were modest, whereas reduction of impulsivity was much more consistent. It has long been observed that low-dose neuroleptics target impulsive symptoms (Coccaro 1998; Soloff 2000). In view of their side effects, however, most particularly the danger of tardive dyskinesia, psychiatrists have been rightly cautious about prescribing these agents. Studies of haloperidol (Cornelius et al. 1993; Soloff et al. 1993; see Table 8–1) have been particularly discouraging, because patients tend to stop taking it and because short-term effects are not found to have been maintained at 6-month follow-up evaluations. In recent years, atypical neuroleptics such as risperidone (Risperdal) and olanzapine, with their milder side effect profiles, have become available. A controlled trial of olanzapine in BPD (Zanarini and Frankenburg 2001) shows that these agents can be used in the same way as older neuroleptics.

Selective serotonin reuptake inhibitors (SSRIs) have been widely used for BPD, usually with the aim of targeting depression. Paradoxically, these agents are much more effective for impulsive symptoms (Coccaro and Kavoussi 1997). (A recent report by Rinne et al. [2002] is an exception to this rule.) High doses of SSRIs (e.g., 60–80 mg of fluoxetine) have a specific effect that reduces self-mutilation (Markowitz 1995), paralleling the use of higher doses for other impulsive disorders (Fava 1997). Controlled trials of SSRIs in BPD have documented modest improvements in mood that fail to match the dramatic effects of antidepressants in melancholic depression.

As documented in Table 8–1, the effects of mood stabilizers are equally modest. The one controlled study of lithium (Links et al. 1990) yielded undramatic results, and results for other mood stabilizers (carbamazepine, valproate, lamotrigine) have been inconsistent and equivocal (Hollander et al. 2001; Soloff 2000). An open trial of sodium valproex (Kavoussi and Coccaro 1998) observed strong anti-impulsive (and weak antidepressant) effects. More research is needed on these agents in large samples to determine whether they are effective in personality disorders. Given the available evidence, the mood stabilizers developed for bipolar mood disorder do not seem to specifically target affective instability in BPD. Instead, like so many other pharmacological agents, mood stabilizers are much more effective in controlling impulsive behavior in patients with BPD. This concords with evidence for the efficacy of valproate in impulsive children with conduct disorder (Fava 1997).

TABLE 8–1. Double-blind placebo-controlled psychopharmacological trials of selective serotonin reuptake inhibitors (SSRIs), mood stabilizers, and neuroleptics for patients with borderline personality disorder (BPD)

Authors	Type	Agent	Sample	N	Mood	Impulsivity	Comments
Markowitz 1995	SSRI	Fluoxetine	BPD	17	+	++	Reduced self-cutting
Salzman et al. 1995	SSRI	Fluoxetine	BPD nonpatient volunteers	27	+	++	
Coccaro and Kavoussi 1997	SSRI	Fluoxetine	BPD with impulsive aggression	40	+	++	
Rinne et al. 2002	SSRI	Fluvoxamine	BPD	38	+	–	
Cowdry and Gardner 1988	Mood stabilizer	Carbamazepine	BPD	16	NS	NS	
Hollander et al. 2001	Mood stabilizer	Divalproex	BPD	12	+	+	High dropout rate
Cowdry and Gardner 1988	Neuroleptic	Trifluoperazine	BPD		+	+	High dropout rate
Soloff et al. 1993	Neuroleptic	Haloperidol	BPD		–	–	High dropout rate
Zanarini and Frankenburg 2001	Neuroleptic	Olanzapine	BPD	28	+	–	6-month study

Note.   – = no response; + = modest response; ++ = strong response; NS = not stated

Thus, pharmacological interventions have not been shown to be useful for *affective instability*, one of the key features of BPD. As shown in a recent study (Koenigsberg et al. 2002), this trait is crucial for distinguishing BPD from other personality disorders. The assumption behind the use of mood stabilizers is that mood changes are essentially the same as those seen in bipolar disorder. However, patients with bipolar disorder do not show changes in mood that vary from hour to hour, depending on interpersonal events. Affective instability in personality disorders may be an entirely different phenomenon with its own unique biology.

Psychopharmacology certainly has a place in treatment regimens for BPD. We have several agents that modulate the most serious forms of impulsive behavior. At present, however, none of the drugs in our armamentarium is specifically effective against the core of borderline pathology. Most patients receiving medication continue to be dysphoric and to have chaotic relationships.

Clinicians may deal with the frustration associated with the partial effectiveness of existing drugs by adding new agents. The result, as shown in a study by Zanarini et al. (2001), is that nearly every patient with BPD ends up being treated with polypharmacy, receiving at least *four or five* drugs (usually one from each class).

Some clinicians have defended the use of polypharmacy because it is based on the idea of separately targeting each dimension of the disorder. We can see this approach in published algorithms for the treatment of BPD (Soloff 2000). Diagrams illustrating algorithms for pharmacological agents appear prominently in the guidelines published by the APA (Oldham et al. 2001). The algorithmic method is standard in psychopharmacology and has been usefully applied to psychoses and mood disorders. As pointed out by critics in the *Journal of Personality Disorders* (McGlashan 2002; Tyrer 2002), however, although these pictures are visually attractive, they do not stand on a firm ground of evidence. When we have little data of limited quality, algorithms can be premature and misleading.

In my view, pharmacological agents are vastly overused in BPD. Sometimes, patients with BPD are given other diagnoses to justify a drug regimen. Patients may be given antidepressants for their "major depression," neuroleptics on the assumption they are psychotic, mood stabilizers if they are seen as having bipolar disorder, or stimulants when their pathology is diagnosed as adult attention-deficit hyperactivity disorder. (For a clinical vignette illustrating these issues, see Example 2 in the section on BPD in Chapter 10) Even when the correct Axis II diagnosis has been made, psychiatrists still feel the need to treat "comorbid" disorders.

Severe substance abuse may have to be treated before personality issues can be addressed. When depression coexists with BPD, the best that can be said for drugs is that they provide marginal relief. As the table documents, effects on mood are surprisingly modest. Moreover, as has been shown in studies of the treatment of depression (Shea et al. 1990), antidepressants do not have the same efficacy in patients with personality disorders as they do in patients without Axis II pathology.

In my opinion, what patients with BPD need most is psychotherapy. In spite of all the doubts and caveats recorded in this chapter, psychological interventions are as well documented for efficacy as any drug. The only reason they are not more extensively used is their cost.

Other Methods of Treatment for Personality Disorders

Most of the research on the treatment of personality disorders has focused on individual psychotherapy and medication. Most clinicians rely on this combination, but these are not the only options. Other therapies described in the literature have a more social dimension: day treatment, milieu therapy, rehabilitation, group therapy, and family therapy. Although there is not much data on these options, they are frequently used in practice, so I briefly examine them here. Because most of this literature concerns BPD, I refer the reader to Gunderson's (2001) clinical guide for details.

Day treatment is a well-established way to treat a wide range of patients with personality disorders, including BPD. Controlled trials on a mixed population of Axis II disorders (Piper et al. 1996) and on patients with BPD (Bateman and Fonagy 1999) have produced encouraging results.

We do not know the precise mechanism by which day treatment works. These programs combine many types of intervention, including individual sessions, group therapy, family therapy, and psychopharmacology. Duration of therapy is another factor: The day programs examined in the randomized controlled trials by Piper et al. and by Bateman and Fonagy lasted at least 6 months. Over this period, improvement could occur through the therapeutic effects of a milieu and/or social and occupational rehabilitation.

Group therapy for personality disorders has been the subject of research. The modality can be used either as a primary method of treatment or as an adjunct to other treatments. In BPD, one trial compared long-term group therapy with individual therapy and found that the two achieve similar results (Munroe-Blum 1992). In another report from the same group (Munroe-Blum and Marziali 1995), patients with BPD had improved function after a course of short-term group therapy. Although these methods have not been examined through randomized controlled trials, they are probably useful, usually in combination with individual therapy.

Family therapy has also been used for patients with personality disorders. Whereas parents were formerly held responsible when a child developed a personality disorder, today's approaches focus on helping families deal with their difficult children. Gunderson has developed a program of psychoeducation for families of patients with BPD, paralleling previous work on expressed emotion in schizophrenia. Gunderson (2001) presented preliminary findings in his book but has not yet published systematic data on the effectiveness of his approach.

Does Treatment Influence Long-Term Outcome?

Whenever I have presented findings about the outcome for personality disorders, one question almost sure to be raised by the audience: Clinicians want to know whether the time they spend with these difficult patients makes a real difference. The question of treatment effectiveness is not a burning question in relation to patients with ASPD, because they rarely remain long in the mental health system, but it is an important issue for patients with BPD, in whom psychotherapists can invest years of effort.

To address this question with any precision, we need large-scale research. The ideal study would be a randomized clinical trial of a specific method of treatment monitoring patients over many years. This option has so far been impractical, in view of the expense and of the high likelihood of noncompliance among populations with personality disorders. We can only make educated guesses about treatment, which should be at least consistent with the findings of naturalistic follow-up studies.

In the absence of randomized controlled trials, it is always difficult to separate naturalistic improvement from true treatment effects. It has been demonstrated that therapy can relieve the worst symptoms of BPD. It is also possible that treatment can sometimes prevent more serious sequelae. However, it has not been shown that any form of therapy consistently leads to full recovery. By and large, results are most impressive in the short term and uncertain in the long term.

The crucial issue is that no one has monitored patients with BPD treated in these trials for more than a year after the completion of treatment. Sadly, Marsha Linehan's original cohort, whose therapy took place in the late 1980s, has never been reevaluated. (Although such research is difficult to fund, our 27-year follow-up was conducted without a grant.)

One of the most striking findings of research on the long-term outcome of BPD is that patients from a variety of social backgrounds, receiving every possible form of treatment (ranging from psychoanalysis to no treatment at all), end, more or less, in the same place. This suggests that time and maturation may ultimately be more important than treatment.

This conclusion, even if it is correct, need not lead us to therapeutic nihilism. Clinical work often involves managing chronicity and sustaining people in the community. Helping people to cope with disabilities is a legitimate, even noble endeavor. Schizophrenia and bipolar disorder are also chronic conditions. Every clinician sees these patients, but few avoid treating them.

The treatment of personality disorders must take individual differences between patients into account. The best results probably emerge in higher-functioning patients. For the more severely ill patients, if therapy can reduce the complications of personality disorders and make naturalistic recovery proceed more rapidly, then the investment of resources is well justified.

9

Suicide and Borderline
Personality Disorder

In this chapter I focus on the difference between acute and chronic suicidality. Again, this crucial issue is greatly illuminated by the findings of outcome research. In the short run, suicidal threats, overdoses, and self-mutilation function as communications of distress. Yet these are not the times when patients are most at risk. Patients with borderline personality disorder (BPD) commit suicide later in the course of their illness, after having lost all hope for recovery.

I also review here data on litigation after completed suicide, to determine the extent to which "defensive medicine" should guide management. I examine whether hospitalization actually prevents suicide in patients with BPD and comment on some of the dangers of admission. Finally, I suggest clinical guidelines for managing chronic suicidality in outpatient treatment.

Acute and Chronic Suicidality

Patients with BPD are chronically suicidal. Frequently, and sometimes continuously, they experience suicidal thoughts. Suicide attempts, in one form or other, occur regularly. Understandably, therapists worry that their patients with BPD will commit suicide. As we have seen, 10% do eventually kill themselves. Yet in the long run, we cannot predict which patients will and which will not.

The term *suicidality* is misleading. It conflates situations in which patients express distress through suicidal gestures and actions with situations in which patients take their own lives. In a landmark study, Maris (1981) found that suicide completers and suicide attempters are, in spite of some degree of overlap, distinct clinical populations. Completers tend to be older, to be male, to use more lethal methods, and to die on the first at-tempt. Attempters tend to be younger, to be female, to use less lethal meth-ods, and to survive.

Some attempters become chronically suicidal, developing what Maris called a "suicidal career." Although the majority stop these behaviors after the first few attempts, their threats cannot be easily dismissed, because Rus-sian roulette can end in death. The chronically suicidal may think about suicide every day for years. Moreover, attempts that are intended to manip-ulate others or to communicate distress can sometimes be fatal.

Thus, therapists have difficulty distinguishing between attempters and completers. Over the last 40 years, suicide attempts have become more fre-quent (Bland et al. 1998), and rates of completed suicide among the young have increased. Therapists often feel particular concern about suicidal ad-olescents. Cases of death by suicide in high school populations have drawn wide publicity. When a 15-year-old threatens suicide, everyone is alarmed. Yet completions prior to the age of 18 are actually quite rare (Blumenthal and Kupfer 1990; Maris 1981). Suicidal adolescents are a highly distressed population, but the vast majority of them remain in the attempter group (Rich et al. 1988).

Chronically suicidal individuals are treatment seeking. In contrast, com-pleters often avoid seeking help. In psychological autopsy studies of youth suicides, Lesage et al. (1994) showed that about one-third met criteria for BPD. However, very few had been in therapy at the time of their death. Less than one-half had seen a mental health professional during the pre-vious year, and one-third had never been evaluated at any point. Similar findings apply to suicide completions at other ages (Bongar et al. 1998).

This suggests the possibility that, compared with suicides in the com-munity, patients in the midst of active treatment represent relatively few suicide completions. We do not see most completers, who either never come for treatment or are seen only briefly, but clinicians remember vividly every suicide in their practice. This gives them a different impression of risk.

In my experience, some suicides can take place at the very beginning of clinical contact with patients with BPD, before an alliance has been estab-lished. As noted in Chapter 5, however, follow-up studies of BPD show that most completions occur late in the course of the illness. Suicides are un-common when patients are in their 20s (when borderline pathology is most dramatic and most frightening). Instead, completions peak in the 30s, when patients are out of treatment, usually after multiple failed attempts at therapy.

Although clinicians should always maintain long-term concern about their patients with BPD, they need not feel high anxiety in the short term. Acute suicidality in BPD, however alarming, should be seen as *a way to com-*

municate distress. The object of this communication can be a significant other, the therapist, or both. Paradoxically, threats of suicide can reflect attachment and involvement in the treatment. Suicide completion, in contrast, is associated with a loss of connection.

Patients with BPD are famous for taking overdoses after quarrels with intimates. As clinicians know, these attempts are "protected"—in the sense that someone has been telephoned, that another person is present when the attempt is made, or that a friend or relative is expected to come by. Occasionally, protection does not work and the patient dies—more by accident than by intention. In most cases, the attempter is saved and brought to the hospital.

Therapists should try to remain calm when a patient with BPD engaged in a treatment makes angry threats, even when accompanied by blood-curdling remarks, such as "You'll read about it in the newspapers." Patients are not as likely to suicide when they are full of anger and tears. If suicidality is a way of communicating distress, then interventions do not necessarily need to protect them against self-destruction but to identify the causes of distress and develop targeted methods of relief from psychic pain.

Self-Mutilation

Not all self-destructive behaviors are lethal. In BPD, parasuicide often takes the form of self-mutilation, one of the most characteristic symptoms of this disorder (Gunderson 2001). Patients with BPD may chronically slash their wrists, as well as other parts of the body. Although these cuts are rarely deep, they are usually repetitive.

Cutting is more easily managed if one keeps in mind that self-mutilation is not really suicidal behavior. Even when covered with scars, patients with BPD do not kill themselves in this way. Cutting is also not predictive of completed suicide (Kroll 1993). Instead, self-mutilation can best be understood as addictive (Linehan 1993). Cutting a wrist translates painful emotions into a relieving flow of blood. Many patients with BPD describe feeling better after cutting, either because dysphoria is relieved, because they feel less numb, or because external pain makes them feel less internal pain (Leibenluft et al. 1987).

Cutting is also a way to communicate. Patients with BPD focus on their negative emotions and act them out in dramatic ways. The purpose is to ensure that others perceive their distress (Zanarini and Frankenburg 1994). If these patients feel no one understands their suffering, their strategy is to turn up the volume. It follows that the management of self-mutilation depends on understanding what each patient is trying to communicate. The focus of interventions should include identifying the emotions behind the act, establishing their causes, and finding better ways of communicating distress.

Suicide and Litigation

Chronic suicidality is draining. Many clinicians have had the experience of not knowing from one week to the next whether a patient will remain alive. To add to the burden, patients with BPD find various ways to anger us, such as missing sessions and then calling at odd hours. It is not surprising that some therapists go out of their way to avoid treating patients with this disorder.

Many therapists have endured completed suicides. Surveys show that death by suicide occurs at least once in the careers of 50% of psychiatrists (Chemtob et al. 1988a) and of 20% of psychologists (Chemtob et al. 1988b), but these are general figures. A clinician treating a selected group of patients in an office practice might avoid losing patients to suicide. At hospital or community clinics, and most particularly in inpatient units, it is hard to find anyone who has never had a patient who committed suicide.

Even one suicide feels like too many. When we have made a major investment in a patient, his or her death leaves us defeated and helpless. As happens with any loss, we feel bereaved, angry, and guilty. These reactions can also lead to an expectation for punishment. To apply a psychodynamic formulation, feelings about suicide or potential suicide can be *projected*. The subject of this projection is often the threat of a lawsuit. For this reason, the fear of litigation can be powerful enough to shape clinical decisions.

This does not mean that lawsuits never happen. (As the saying goes, even paranoids have enemies.) In spite of their best intentions, therapists can be sued. Suicide is the leading cause of lawsuits against mental health professionals, accounting for 20% of cases (Kelley 1996). Although I have never had personal experience with lawsuits, I know from colleagues about the suffering litigation can bring.

How frequently do families sue therapists after suicide? And how often are such suits upheld in the courts? On the basis of data drawn from various jurisdictions around the United States (Bongar et al. 1998; Gutheil 1992), it appears that only a very small fraction of suicides occurring in the course of treatment lead to litigation. Moreover, only a minority (about 20%) of lawsuits against mental health clinicians are eventually upheld. Thus, most practitioners will never have to endure a lawsuit, and most of those who do will win the case.

In Canada, where I practice, people tend to be less litigious than they are in the United States (at least in certain regions). North of the border, lawsuits after suicide are uncommon and usually unsuccessful. A systematic study (Beilby 2000) showed that of 255 suits against psychiatrists in Canada over a 9-year period in the past decade, 53 (21%) followed a suicide or a suicide attempt. Of these, 90% led to judgments in favor of the clinician (Fine and Sansone 1990; Maltsberger 1994). Psychiatrists were found liable only in 6 cases. In a country of 25 million people, judgments against clinicians who lose a patient to suicide occur once every 2 years.

What is the basis of a lawsuit that claims negligence? The plaintiff must show that the clinician failed to meet an accepted "standard of care" and that the negligence was a "proximate cause" of the death (Kelley 1996). In other words, the therapist must have failed to provide a degree of care that a reasonably prudent person or professional should exercise in the same or similar circumstances, and this error must have been a direct cause of the outcome.

Failing to predict suicide does not, by itself, constitute negligence. Lawsuits in which clinicians are found liable have not been based on the fact of suicide alone (Bongar 1992; Kelley 1996). Rather, liability depends on clinical misjudgment, most particularly the failure to assess patients carefully and the absence of adequate clinical records documenting the clinician's rationale for management. Thus, courts understand that suicide cannot always be prevented and do not routinely hold clinicians responsible when it happens. It is another story if a patient's condition has never been properly assessed or if detailed medical records of evaluations have not been kept.

The vast majority of lawsuits after suicide involve inpatients, with only a small fraction of cases from outpatient treatment. Most concern not whether the patient should have been hospitalized in the first place but whether the patient was discharged too early. Finally, litigation usually involves patients being treated for major Axis I disorders. Very few concern patients with chronic suicidality.

Bongar et al. (1998) described a series of common "failure" scenarios corresponding to these principles. Twelve circumstances are most likely to lead to litigation after suicide:

1. Failure to evaluate the need for pharmacotherapy
2. Failure to evaluate the need for hospitalization (i.e., not establishing and documenting a rationale for maintaining outpatient therapy)
3. Failure to maintain boundaries in the relationship with the patient
4. Failures in supervision and consultation
5. Failure to evaluate suicidality at intake
6. Failure to evaluate suicidality at management transitions
7. Failure to obtain a good history or to obtain prior records
8. Failure to conduct a mental status

9. Failure in diagnosis
10. Failure to establish formal treatment plan
11. Failure to make the environment safe (e.g., removing pills or weapons)
12. Failure to document clinical judgments, rationales, and observations

These scenarios also suggest that a well-thought-out clinical plan and careful recordkeeping can define competent clinical practice. It does *not* follow that suicidal patients must routinely be hospitalized. If patients nonetheless commit suicide, the therapist's legal position will be defensible.

Litigation can be an outcome of the anger of relatives. Families who are dealing with the same feelings about patients that we experience may be tempted to make us the scapegoat for suicide (Kelley 1996). Therefore, involving the family in treatment can make lawsuits after suicide less likely. As Hoge et al. (1989, p. 619) state, "It is an axiom among malpractice attorneys that clinicians who maintain good relationships with their patients do not get sued." Although this principle cannot apply to a dead patient, it does apply to establishing relationships with families of suicidal patients. Usually, contact will be established with the consent of the patient, but when the patient is in danger, the family should always be consulted. If they are not, bereaved relatives have every right to be angry.

Packman and Harris (1998) recommended that therapists inform suicidal patients early in treatment that their families will be contacted if they are seen to be at risk. I would go even further. A therapist treating a chronically suicidal patient should make a point of talking to relatives and significant others at an early stage. This practice need not involve any breach of confidentiality. It parallels the relationships we have with the families of patients with psychoses and other severe illnesses.

These contacts can also be clinically useful, because we can gain information about the patient that might not otherwise be available. However, the main goal of seeing relatives is to inform them of the rationale behind the treatment, to educate them about the clinician's management plan, and to obtain their cooperation with the therapy. Family members themselves have had to endure the patient's chronic suicidality. Bringing them into an alliance is supportive. It may also help protect the therapist from being held responsible for an unfavorable outcome.

Finally, when suicides do occur, therapists can conduct a "postvention" (Bongar 1992). In other words, they should meet with the family soon after the death of the patient. Again, there is no breach of confidentiality, because we need not reveal the patient's secrets. Postvention allows the clinician to deal empathically with bereaved relatives and to help the family with the consequences of a loss.

Is Suicide Prevention Possible?

Clinicians are trained to recognize suicidality and to use it to guide their interventions. Yet there is a surprising lack of empirical evidence demonstrating that treatment actually prevents patients from completing suicide. This is not only the case for personality disorders; it has been difficult to demonstrate that admitting patients with *any* psychiatric diagnosis prevents suicide.

The reason is that suicide in patients with mental disorders is not really predictable. It is difficult to predict or prevent rare events (Goldstein et al. 1991; Pokorny 1983). Even when we identify factors associated with a higher risk and when (particularly in large samples) such associations are found to be statistically significant, it proves impossible to predict suicide in any single case. Algorithms used to guide suicide prediction yield too many false positives to be clinically useful.

How then should we assess the enormous effort that has gone into suicide prevention? Many initiatives have been introduced over the years, and one would expect them to have had an impact on prevalence by now. Yet in spite of the vastly increased availability of mental health services, overall suicide rates in North America have remained steady and, until recently, were increasing in young adult populations (Sudak et al. 1984). Compared with the mid-twentieth century, our society is blessed with a vast increase in psychotherapists. Yet more young people than ever are committing suicide.

One way of testing the effectiveness of interventions is to compare the prevalence of suicide where services are available with the prevalence where they are not. In England, a telephone contact organization called the Samaritans was developed as a preventive method. Shortly after these services were introduced, suicide rates did go down. However, later research suggested the reduction was more likely due to a concurrent event: decreased availability of a lethal method (inhaling toxic gas from cooking stoves). To test specifically whether the Samaritans had played a role in lowering rates, a controlled study (Jennings et al. 1978) compared communities in which contact was available and those in which it was not. No difference in the frequency of completions was found. By and large, although hotlines provide service to the people who call them, there is no evidence that they prevent suicide.

It has long been shown that therapy can reduce the frequency of suicide *attempts* (Sudak et al. 1984). Yet in the entire literature, only a few reports seriously suggest that treatment reduces completion. Most of these findings come from Scandinavia and concern the treatment of classical mood disorders. In bipolar disorder, patients who continue taking lithium are less likely to die by suicide than those who do not (Nilsson 1999). Moreover, suicide rates have fallen as antidepressant prescriptions have become more common (Isacsson et al. 1996; Ohberg et al. 1998). A program to educate physicians about depression in a Swedish community lowered the suicide rate within a year (Rihmer et al. 1995; Rutz 2001). In this study, the prevalence rebounded to the same level by 2-year follow-up evaluation, but local physicians who received training might have been providing better service to depressed patients, treating them at an earlier stage before they became suicidal.

Yet it is difficult to be certain that relationships between intervention and completion are truly causal. Patients with more severe bipolar illness may be less compliant with lithium treatment. Scandinavian suicide rates, which have traditionally been high, may be declining for other reasons. The study in which physicians were trained to recognize suicidality needs replication. Nonetheless, it seems likely that better treatment of classical mood disorders can reduce suicide completions.

These findings need not apply to patients with personality disorders who are chronically suicidal. In this population, where treatment is much more arduous, it does not seem likely that community programs focusing on rapid intervention would have the same impact. Unlike depression, where drug therapy can be strikingly effective, chronically suicidal patients with personality disorders do not obtain dramatic benefits from pharmacological treatment.

Does Hospitalization Prevent Suicide in BPD?

I have often heard colleagues state that treatment decisions for suicidal patients must be based on *safety*. In practice, this usually implies that patients who threaten suicide require hospitalization. Some even believe that denying a suicidal patient admission to hospital constitutes malpractice.

Hospital admission for suicide threats is recommended in the American Psychiatric Association's *Practice Guidelines for the Treatment of Borderline Personality Disorder* (American Psychiatric Association 2001). As a consultant in this process, I wrote to the committee to point out the lack of any supporting evidence for this suggestion but was unable to influence the final draft.

In my opinion, hospital admission is most useful in an *acute* situation. No one would doubt the importance of hospitalizing suicidal patients with melancholic or psychotic depression, particularly in the absence of a personality disorder. The efficacy of treatment methods in such cases (i.e., antidepressants and/or electroconvulsive therapy) is well established, with good results common within a few weeks (Elkin et al. 1989).

In contrast, the management of *chronic* suicidality must be based on different principles (Fine and Sansone 1990; Maltsberger 1994). Neither biological treatments nor other short-term interventions provide a quick fix for the problem. Moreover, as shown by follow-up studies, patients with BPD, unlike those with melancholic or psychotic depression, hardly ever suicide while hospitalized and rarely do so immediately after being discharged.

Under what conditions are patients with BPD admitted to a hospital? Hull et al. (1996) documented the most common scenarios: 1) psychotic episodes, 2) serious suicide attempts, 3) suicidal threats, and 4) self-mutilation. Let us consider them one by one.

The logic in admitting patients for a brief psychosis is that we have a specific treatment (i.e., neuroleptics) that can control symptoms. The admission of patients after life-threatening suicide attempts also has some value. At the very least, such circumstances require giving a break to family and to the outpatient therapist. Even if no active treatment is conducted in the hospital, admission provides an opportunity to assess precipitating factors and review the treatment plan.

It is a different story when clinicians admit patients with BPD for suicidal threats or for self-mutilation, particularly when these patients are hospitalized repeatedly. Aggressive attempts at suicide prevention under these circumstances, particularly when they involve frequent and lengthy hospitalizations, have never been shown to be effective.

Are these interventions cost-effective? The resources required for inpatient treatment are very expensive. I believe they should be used for specific treatment plans that can be carried out only in a hospital. Pharmacotherapy for psychosis and for severe mood disorders are good examples, but for the hospitalized patient with BPD, there may be no such plan. Instead, admission may provide nothing but a suicide watch. If, as so often happens, the patient becomes suicidal again shortly after discharge, little has been accomplished.

Some experts (e.g., Kernberg 1976) have proposed that hospitalization can make it possible to carry out psychotherapy, by allowing time to establish a therapeutic alliance. However, no empirical evidence supports this argument. No one has ever carried out a controlled trial showing that psychotherapy is more effective in a hospital setting. In any case, managed care has vastly restricted this option.

Chronic suicidal ideation "goes with the territory" of BPD. These symptoms remit only late in the course of treatment. Clinicians treating patients with BPD have to accept chronic suicidality and get on with the job of treating its causes.

Negative Effects of Hospitalization in Borderline Personality Disorder

Safety is a buzzword. Who could possibly be against it? The problem is that this use of language finesses an empirical question. Is the suicidal patient with BPD actually safer in a hospital?

Hospitalization is a two-edged sword. Procedures developed for acute suicidality in mood disorders are rarely appropriate for chronic suicidality. Most clinicians recognize the scenario in which patients with BPD escalate suicidal or self-mutilating behaviors while hospitalized. Two mechanisms help account for this phenomenon. First, for patients with poor social supports, a week in a ward or even a night in an emergency department, provides a reinforcing level of social contact. Second, the environment of a psychiatric ward acts as a reinforcer, because patients who cut themselves or who carry out parasuicidal actions receive more, not less, nursing care.

Thus, hospitalization sometimes reinforces the very suicidal behaviors that therapists are trying to extinguish. Linehan (1993), applying the principles of behavioral psychology, discouraged admission for precisely this reason and was willing to tolerate only an overnight "hold." Dawson and MacMillan (1993) took an even more radical position, arguing that we should *never* hospitalize these patients. Perhaps one should never say "never," but clinicians should be at least be aware of the dangers of admitting chronically suicidal patients.

A patient who eventually recovered from BPD described her experiences in an article in *Psychiatric Services*, which included the following admonition:

> Do not hospitalize a person with borderline personality disorder for more than 48 hours. My self-destructive episodes—one leading right into another—came out only after my first and subsequent hospital admissions, after I learned the system was usually obligated to respond.... When you as a service provider do not give the expected response to these threats, you'll be accused of not caring. What you are really doing is being cruel to be kind. When my doctor wouldn't hospitalize me, I accused him of not caring if I lived or died. He replied, referring to a cycle of repeated hospitalizations, "That's not life." And he was 100 percent right! (Williams 1998, p. 174)

When treatment of BPD does spiral out of control, therapists need the help of a specialized team. The decision to hospitalize a patient may sometimes be a consequence of a lack of alternative resources, either in a crisis team or in a day hospital. To handle these situations, partial hospitalization in a day treatment center may be a particularly useful option. Effectiveness has been empirically demonstrated in two different patient cohorts (Bateman and Fonagy 1999; Piper et al. 1996). Unfortunately, no one has conducted a parallel study of full hospitalization. Nor has anyone conducted a study comparing the effectiveness of day hospital treatment with that of full admission.

Partial hospitalization may be particularly effective for patients with BPD. Day hospitals offer a highly structured program. When activities are scheduled every hour, little time remains to slash one's wrists. Regression is further limited by the fact that the patient goes home at night. (In the absence of evidence that full hospitalization prevents suicide completion, it makes sense to tolerate this degree of risk.)

Management of Suicidality in Outpatient Settings

I strongly favor outpatient management of BPD. My approach is described in detail in Chapter 10. But how can clinicians handle suicide threats in these settings? Following principles developed by Linehan (1993), one first must conduct a *behavioral analysis*. This involves listening to the emotional content of suicidality and validating the dysphoric feelings that tempt the patient to act out impulsively. A second step involves identifying the circumstances leading the patient to have these feelings. The third step is to establish a dialogue with the patient to develop alternative solutions to these precipitating problems. Essentially, the cognitive-behavioral approach involves strategies to increase emotion tolerance, to decenter emotions, and to modify cognitive appraisals.

More specifically, when patients threaten suicide, the therapist should respond empathically, commenting on how intolerable dysphoric emotions must be for death to be an option. The dialogue then moves on to an understanding of what brought on these feelings and to implementing strategies to reduce their intensity. The last step involves problem-solving, which offers practical alternatives to the all-or-nothing thinking that is associated with suicidality (Schneidman 1981).

Therapists managing BPD also set up a hierarchy of goals for different traits, corresponding to the underlying dimensions of the disorder described by Siever and Davis (1991). This strategic framework has been recommended in clinical guides to treatment by Linehan (1993) and Gunderson (2001). Impulsivity has to be the first target, because acting out prevents therapy from addressing other goals. Once the patient is calm enough to work on treatment, the focus shifts to the modification of affective instability.

Ultimately, excessive focus on preventing suicide completion prevents therapists from doing their job. Treatment has to help patients to solve problems. When we spend all our time worrying about suicide completion, the therapeutic process is derailed. We need to maintain a focus on the task at hand and to understand suicide threats as communications of distress. For this reason, therapists who treat patients with BPD need thick skins! We need to let clients know that we hear them and that we are aware of their suffering. At the same time, we need to get on with the task of therapy. Maintaining one's *sangfroid* in the face of suicidal threats is easier said than done but may be the only way to make progress.

When therapy begins to work, suicidality often drops out of the clinical picture. The explanation is commonsensical: When patients feel empowered, they have no further reason to choose death. Ultimately, patients with BPD remain suicidal for long periods of time because they do not feel in control of their lives. In other words, they actually *need* to be suicidal (Fine and Sansone 1990). If one has no power over life, one can still have the power to choose death. From this point of view, we should be cautious about removing this useful coping mechanism too soon. For some patients, only the knowledge that they can die allows them to go on living.

10

Working With Traits

This chapter suggests an approach to treatment that takes the precursors, course, and outcome of personality disorders into account. The key principles are to accept chronicity and to concentrate on rehabilitation.

I describe here a general model of treatment and then apply it to the modification of traits commonly seen in personality disorders, focusing on three clinically important categories: borderline, narcissistic, and avoidant. Five clinical examples are presented to illustrate how the model works in practice.

The reader should be aware of some caveats. I do not claim that my ideas about psychotherapy are unique. Nor have I proven that my approach is effective. In previous chapters, I criticized others for basing the treatment of personality disorders on clinical experience rather than on empirical data, and I should apply the same standards to myself. However, therapists treating patients with personality disorders do not yet have a solid evidence base on which to conduct practice. My recommendations aim to be practical and to be at least consistent with existing research.

Therapy for personality disorders stands on three general principles. First, because personality traits are stable over time, we need not attempt to achieve radical change. It is sufficient to help patients to reach a better level of functioning. Second, the chronic course of personality disorders implies that we must set realistic goals. Therefore, expectations from therapy must be scaled down and small gains seen as significant victories. Third, patients need to focus not on the past but on the way they feel, think, and behave in the present. In this light, the model that makes the most sense for treating personality disorders is cognitive-behavioral therapy.

Trait Modification in Personality Disorders

It is illusory to expect therapy to change personality, but traits can be modified in ways that affect their behavioral expression. Moreover, patients can learn to make more judicious and selective use of existing traits. The same characteristics that are maladaptive in some contexts can be adaptive in other contexts. Therefore, patients can capitalize on strong points by selecting environments in which traits are most likely to be useful. They can also minimize weak points by avoiding environments in which their traits are not useful.

I described this approach in an earlier book, *Working with Traits* (Paris 1998b). I expand on those ideas here, placing them in the context of chronicity, course, and outcome.

To understand how to treat patients with personality disorders, we might first consider how they improve naturalistically, without treatment. This trajectory is most striking in impulsive disorders. As we have seen, recovery comes from modulating problematical behaviors and finding more adaptive solutions to problems. The goal of therapy is to speed up this process.

Psychotherapy is a form of education. In personality disorders, the curriculum consists of showing patients how to make better and more adaptive use of traits. Formal teaching takes place in the therapist's office. Life outside the sessions is the laboratory. Learning and applying new behaviors to old situations is the homework.

The general model of treatment for personality disorders can be divided into four steps:

1. *Identifying* when traits or behavioral patterns are maladaptive
2. *Observing* the emotional states that lead to problematic behaviors
3. *Experimenting* with more effective alternatives to see how they work
4. *Practicing* new strategies

Let us now see how this approach can be applied to the traits most associated with personality pathology.

Impulsivity

High levels of impulsivity carry a risk for a wide range of mental disorders. Yet impulsive traits can also be adaptive. In conditions of great danger, a rapid response may be lifesaving. The problem is to know when to act fast and when to step back and carefully consider a situation.

Impulsive individuals can benefit from choosing environments in which action is a virtue. Ideally, they should find work in which rapid responses are useful (e.g., law enforcement or hospital emergency departments). Needless to say, even in these environments, one must harness impulses and use judgment. Impulsive individuals can also avoid environments in which rapid responses are a palpable handicap (e.g., routine work in an office or a factory). Not everyone has a choice of employment, but even when forced into an occupation that is irremediably predictable, impulsive people can express their traits by taking up sublimatory activities (such as sky diving or car racing).

Impulsivity is particularly likely to create problems in close interpersonal relationships. Intimacy is the greatest challenge most people face in life. Many succeed at everything *except* intimate relationships. It takes enormous flexibility to manage the complexities of being and remaining in love. As we have seen, patients with borderline personality disorder (BPD) have great trouble with intimacy and sometimes do better by avoiding it. When involved with another person on a long-term basis, they should choose a less impulsive partner to rein them in.

Research shows that successful marital choices depend on similarities. Stability of marriage is predicted by commonalities in social background and physical appearance (Bird and Melville 1994). However, stable partners need not necessarily share similar personality traits. Instead, as suggested many years ago by Dicks (1967), marriages do best when both people have comparable levels of overall functioning but have *complementary* (rather than supplementary) personality profiles. A good example of this principle is the well-known "compulsive-histrionic pairing" (Jacobsen and Gurman 1995), in which the emotional control of one partner balances the expressiveness of the other.

In contrast, two impulsive individuals in one relationship make an explosive mixture. Patients with BPD are sometimes attracted to individuals with antisocial or narcissistic traits (Paris and Braverman 1995). These are people who, at least initially, make the patient with BPD feel wanted. Unfortunately, these relationships are highly unstable.

Impulsive traits must be modulated by clear and predictable structures. In intimate relationships, boundaries can be provided by a well-grounded partner. Thus, when patients with BPD marry, they may do better to choose spouses who can function as caretakers (Paris and Braverman 1995).

Affective Lability

Emotionality can be an asset or a problem (Beck and Freeman 1990). At their best, affectively labile individuals are lively, stimulating, and empathic. At their worst, they are mercurial and unstable.

Affectively labile individuals may benefit from settings in which intense emotional responses are a virtue. Emotionality, in combination with what trait psychologists call extraversion and openness to experience, is associated with being a "people person." Thus, occupations that involve working directly with the public may provide suitable settings for people who are oriented toward others and talented in communication. Affectively labile people may even be attracted to the practice of psychotherapy, but to succeed in this kind of work, they must learn how to modulate their responses (Paris 1981).

Emotional intensity is particularly likely to be a problem in intimate relationships. As research on marriage has shown (Gottman and Levenson 2000), persistent negative tone in a couple relationship is a strong long-term predictor of divorce. Lovers quarrel—but to maintain a stable relationship, one has to take time out, calm down, and try again. This is more difficult for affectively unstable individuals, who tend to be aroused easily and who take longer to return to baseline. Therefore, people with these traits are best advised to seek out partners who are less emotional than themselves. Again, the "compulsive-histrionic" pair (Jacobsen and Gurman 1995) tends to be more stable—even if the compulsive partner complains about excessive emotional demands and even if the histrionic partner complains about unresponsiveness and distance.

Anxiety

Anxious traits can also be adaptive or maladaptive (Beck and Freeman 1990). When one is faced with an ambiguous and novel situation, or when the outside world is actually dangerous, standing back from the fray or withdrawing can be the best strategy. Problems arise when anxiety interferes with learning the essential skills for social interaction (Kagan 1994). In the modern world, personal autonomy is increasingly essential for success, both in love and in work.

People with anxious traits need a predictable environment. They may therefore be best advised to choose occupations that reward careful, slow, and persistent work. Classic examples in which one can observe useful compulsive traits include accountants, secretaries, and physicians.

The most common problem for individuals with anxious traits involves their difficulty establishing relationships and intimacy. In my experience, some choose a partner who is less anxious and "brings them out," whereas others are more comfortable with people like themselves. In either case, anxious individuals need to develop a secure and stable social network, making use of contact with and support from a few reliable people.

Borderline Personality Disorder

In BPD, therapy requires the modification of two underlying traits: impulsivity and affective instability. To modulate these characteristics, patients must understand the communicative functions of actions, identify emotional states, and learn alternative ways of handling conflict. These skills are the basic elements in Linehan's (1993) dialectical behavior therapy.

The traits associated with BPD can lead to problems at work or at school. Often, conflicts emerge with supervisors, colleagues, or teachers, who are seen as uncaring or abusive. These perceptions are filtered through all-or-nothing cognitive schema (splitting). These perceptions, typical of patients with BPD, involve seeing the world as made up of people who are either unconditionally loving or totally untrustworthy. The therapist must help these patients to correct such distortions, to see others with normal ambivalence, and to negotiate interpersonal conflicts effectively (Gunderson 2001).

Kroll (1988) emphasized that patients with BPD must, above all, develop *competence*. Gunderson (2001) takes a similar view: Whatever difficulties they have in their intimate lives, these patients need a stable and independent source of self-esteem outside the conflictual arena of interpersonal conflict. Follow-up studies of BPD (McGlashan 1993) show that the ability to work is related to recovery. Once work is stabilized, it becomes easier to deal with the problems of intimacy.

Whatever the working situation, much of the therapy with these patients focuses on problems in intimacy—relationships with lovers, with close friends, and with family members. Patients with BPD are quick to move close to other people—and quick to be disappointed with them. This pattern, once identified, must be modified by learning to slow down emotionally when one meets new people and to take the necessary time to assess their good and bad qualities. Eventually, patients with BPD can also learn how to absorb the inevitable disappointments associated with any close relationship.

Impulsivity in BPD is closely related to suicidality, the most troubling problem in this population. Yet, as discussed in Chapter 9, we should not be driven by fear. Suicidality has to be tolerated because it is the way the patient with BPD communicates distress. The therapist should respond to suicidal thoughts and behaviors as communications to be understood rather than threats to be acted on. Thus, when patients slash their wrists, the therapist should spend more time talking about distress and less time on cutting. Similarly, after an overdose of pills, once medical treatment has been carried out, the therapist should quickly resume the tasks of therapy and explore the circumstances leading up to the attempt. This approach does not ignore suicidality. Rather, it concentrates on what the patient is trying to say through such behaviors. Instead of letting the threat of suicide dominate the agenda, this approach keeps therapy in a problem-solving mode.

Patients with BPD have a broad range of other impulsive behaviors. They may abuse substances, be sexually promiscuous, or have tantrums in which they destroy property. In each of these situations, the task of the therapist is much the same—to identify underlying emotions and to examine in what alternative way the patient might have handled the dysphoria.

Impulsivity in BPD is associated with behaviors that interfere with the process of therapy. Some, such as severe substance abuse, may have to be controlled before other treatments can take place (Gunderson 2001). Other common "therapy-interfering behaviors" (Linehan 1993) can include coming late and missing sessions entirely. At high levels of impulsivity, therapy becomes impossible. The patient needs to know there are limits beyond which treatment may have to be discontinued.

The other aspect of treating BPD involves learning how to modulate affective instability. Therapists who work with patients with BPD know how to empathize with highly dysphoric feelings, even when they are far from ordinary experience. These patients are famous for their anger but are just as likely to be chronically depressed and anxious. Accepting and working with these emotions is an implicit "holding environment."

Helping patients with BPD to manage dysphoric emotions is a central element of any treatment. *Short-range* strategies include distraction, decentering, and reappraisal. Each patient has to learn on an individual basis what works best when he or she is upset. *Long-range* strategies involve identifying and solving the problems that produce these emotions. The crucial point is to learn that there are ways, other than impulsive actions, to relieve dysphoria.

Example 1

Presentation

Angela was a 25-year-old graduate student who complained of suicidal ideas, self-mutilation, and intermittent voices in her head telling her to kill herself. She was having difficulty at school and was experiencing conflict in a love affair.

Angela was involved with Mario, with whom she shared interests in politics, literature, and music. Mario found Angela to be exciting and unique but had difficulty functioning as the caretaker in the relationship. In particular, he could not handle Angela's self-mutilation. This behavior had become addictive over the years. Originally, cutting had communicated resentment against the insensitivity of her family. More recently, it was linked with jealousy. On two separate occasions, after attending a party, they quarreled over the time Mario spent with another woman. These evenings ended with Angela, fueled by alcohol intake, breaking things in the apartment and slashing her wrists.

Angela had been a well-behaved child who obtained high marks at school. She described her parents as well-meaning but insensitive to her feelings. As an adolescent, Angela upset them by developing a "punk" identity. Unknown to her family, she became sexually promiscuous while abusing a series of substances.

Therapy

Identifying. The first step of therapy involved acknowledging her maladaptive behaviors and recognizing that the problem lay in herself and not in others.

Observing. The second step involved showing Angela how her behaviors were triggered by threatened abandonment, an issue of particular sensitivity.

Experimenting. Each time Angela was tempted to cut her wrists, she was encouraged to examine the feelings leading to the impulse and to consider alternative ways of handling these emotions. Angela was also taught to identify her responses at an early stage, so that she could learn to process them internally before they became overwhelming.

Practicing. By expressing emotions without having to "turn up the volume," Angela would actually be more likely to be heard. She was also encouraged to take "time out" when she noticed her anger getting out of control, so as to return to the issue in a calmer frame of mind.

Over the course of several months, Angela reduced the frequency of self-mutilation. At the same time, the auditory hallucinations, usually brought on by extreme dysphoria, also came under control. The relationship with Mario came to an end. After the breakup, Angela was encouraged to avoid intimacy for a while and to build up a wider social network. Angela concentrated on her thesis, and this work protected her by providing a source of stable self-esteem.

Follow-Up Findings

Angela left the city after finishing her studies. I obtained 10-year follow-up information through a family friend. Angela was followed supportively by another therapist for another year and then was able to discontinue treatment. She became involved in literary circles, publishing stories and poetry. This world, which encouraged strong expression of emotions, allowed her to express emotions without amplifying or acting on them. She married a protective husband from the business community, devoted herself to raising two children, and continued to write.

Example 2

Presentation

Catherine, a 24-year-old nurse, came to therapy with a continuous and intense obsession about suicide. Given her profession, she had ready access to the means for completion. However, in spite of constant threats, she never actually made an attempt. Catherine's impulsivity was also expressed in deeply troubled relationships. She had been intimately involved with a series of antisocial men, even helping to hide them from the police. These liaisons, all of which were tumultuous and unstable, usually involved sexual experimentation and polysubstance abuse.

After a few months of treatment, Catherine was hospitalized for a brief psychotic episode. After visiting her alcoholic father, whom she had not seen in many years, she began to hear voices and believed that the world was coming to an end. This episode resolved within a few days.

Catherine had been an irritable and moody child who obtained little support from the important people in her life. Her mother had died young, and her father had given her up to foster care. Her foster parents raised her with consistent rules and helped Catherine to become a nurse. Yet she could never forgive them for failing to respond to her emotional needs.

Therapy

Identifying.   It took time for Catherine to acknowledge maladaptive patterns. At first, she tried to explain to the therapist why the men in her life were not as bad as they seemed, and how they benefited from her support. Gradually, she developed enough trust to acknowledge the ways in which she was being exploited.

Observing.   Catherine, although often raging within, lacked effective ways to communicate her anger. Instead of getting the men in her life to express emotions for her, she needed to find ways of processing her feelings as well as learn to assert herself. Her failure in self-assertion, apparent at work and in relationships, was based on a fear of being rejected. Typically, she found that angry and sad feelings overwhelmed her, and she would suppress them, creating a kind of emotional fog. Catherine also distracted herself through a long series of exciting and dangerous involvements with men.

Experimenting.   Catherine's therapy focused on learning new strategies to contain dysphoria. She developed self-soothing (reading, music) to replace her former need to spend all her free time with a man. She also took additional professional training and looked for new challenges in her career.

Practicing.   Over the course of the treatment, Catherine learned to avoid dangerous men, replacing them with a stable network of female friends. She learned how to make her work more rewarding, eventually developing a specialty in geriatric nursing.

Follow-Up Findings

Catherine moved away but kept touch with me through Christmas cards. Now 50 years old, she had never married but found satisfaction through friendship, intellectual interests, and her work.

Narcissistic Personality Disorder

Grandiosity is the central characteristic of narcissistic personality disorder (NPD; Gunderson and Ronningstam 2001). This is the trait that gets patients into the most difficulty and that therapy most needs to tame.

Inevitably, life batters down everyone's grandiosity. We must all deal with disappointment and failure and come to terms with limitations. This is the essence of maturity. However, patients with NPD have trouble remaining on this trajectory. When they are young, they often seem attractive and promising. Yet as they age, they are unable to deal with losses, so that their later years are marked by disappointment and bitterness (Kernberg 1987). In spite of their overtly high self-esteem, individuals with NPD tend to crash when they fail.

Torgersen (1995) found that patients with NPD experience a surprisingly high level of dysphoria, largely due to unsatisfactory intimate relationships. They tend to seek treatment after a series of setbacks in intimacy. Torgersen reported that patients with NPD have unstable long-term relationships with a relatively low rate of marriage and a high rate of divorce when they do marry.

People with NPD can be impressive to others. They may speak well and have special talents or qualities. Some are successful at work and have serious difficulties only in intimate relationships, whereas others fail to meet expectations at the workplace. These difficulties are due to a lack of persistence and an inability to collaborate with others. Patients with NPD tend to respond to negative feedback with anger, a reaction that usually makes a bad situation worse. These individuals do not often understand that other people's evaluations are usually valid.

Patients with NPD lack empathy. One primary goal of therapy is to teach these skills. This is not easy, because individuals with low empathy fail to observe how their behavior affects other people. They also present distorted or self-serving versions of events to the therapist. Unless these patients learn to take responsibility for their mistakes, they will continue to make the same ones. This is one reason why therapy for this group is so often ineffective and/or interminable.

Kohut (1970, 1977) claimed that patients with NPD need a highly empathic therapist. His concept of a healing environment is in accord with research findings on the role of nonspecific factors in successful therapy. By itself, however, empathy from a therapist is rarely sufficient to control consistently maladaptive behavior. Often, the most crucial interventions involve demonstrating the *consequences* of narcissistic behavior. These patients require confrontations to identify problem behaviors and to develop adaptive alternatives.

Kohut's approach also included reviewing childhood experiences in which patients with NPD failed to receive empathy from caretakers. Yet his idea that patients with NPD benefit from discovering that their parents did not love them sufficiently is problematic. For these patients, it is all too easy to use a sense of deprivation to support entitlements.

Patients with NPD typically believe that their personality does not need to change very much. Instead, other people should treat them better. Thinking well of oneself without brooding unduly on one's defects can be associated with success in life, but patients come for treatment when these traits stop working for them, usually in their intimate relationships.

Therapists must be cautious about validating the worldview of the narcissist. Usually, we usually lack sufficient information to determine how patients are actually behaving. Like patients with BPD, those with NPD often present the therapist with a distorted picture of their interpersonal world. It takes a good deal of skill to read between the lines and reconstruct what actually happened. Sometimes the picture remains cloudy and can be clarified only by interviewing key informants.

The most difficult problem in treating NPD involves getting patients to identify maladaptive patterns. Tactful confrontations are needed to help these patients perceive and acknowledge problems. They also have to be taught how to see interpersonal conflicts from other people's point of view and to not attribute other people's reactions to neglect or malevolence. These patients are often poor at knowing what other people want and at negotiating compromises so that all parties get to meet some portion of their needs. At the same time, they need to see that self-serving behaviors do not work.

Example 3

Presentation

David was a 28-year-old lawyer who presented with difficulty establishing intimate relationships. Although a good worker, he had continual conflicts with his supervisors, who failed to recognize his unique abilities. David imagined living in a penthouse, surrounded by women and envied by other men, but in real life, he was consistently rejected. David became addicted to pornographic videos and spent money in bars paying strippers to perform. His sense of entitlement also led him to carry out minor crimes. A woman with whom he had a brief love affair had dropped him. He then went to her apartment and stole several items of her jewelry, which he kept around his house. On another occasion, when his own apartment was broken into, he made fraudulent insurance claims that netted him thousands of dollars. On a third occasion, he got into a serious brawl with his younger brother, spending a night in jail before charges were dropped.

David's irritable temperament had been apparent early in life. He was demanding with his parents and physically aggressive with his brothers. These traits became amplified in his adolescence when his parents split up, after which his father became totally unreliable and his mother became impoverished and embittered.

Therapy

Identifying. David was at least partially aware that he was a difficult person. The initial stage of treatment involved helping him to identify maladaptive patterns in which his exploitative behavior led to rejection.

Observing. David needed to learn how to observe his own reactions. Behind his arrogant exterior, he was easily deflated and highly sensitive to approval (or disapproval) by other people.

Experimenting. The first goal of therapy was to stabilize David's work situation. After getting in trouble by rudely contradicting a supervisor at a committee meeting, David realized that, whatever the merits of the case, his behavior was out of line. In a similar incident, he stopped himself from manipulating company records to obtain greater financial rewards.

The second goal focused on improving intimate relationships. David became involved with Carla, a wealthy woman from a prominent family. David imagined leaving the firm to live among the rich and famous, but he remained unskilled in listening and understanding another person. Whenever Carla was preoccupied, either with work, family, or friends, David would become enraged. Their quarrels escalated to the point of becoming physical. Carla retaliated by starting a lesbian affair with a close friend. David had actually suggested at one point that they have a threesome, but when Carla acted first, he felt crushed and excluded.

Practicing. David responded gradually to confrontations as to where he had gone wrong. He came to acknowledge the reason why Carla's lover had displaced him, which was that she was more supportive. He spent the next few months concentrating on his work, staying away from intimate relationships until he could handle them better.

Follow-Up Findings

Five years after therapy ended, I received a call from David, now living in another city. He informed me, to my surprise, that he had married Carla. David explained that they had both matured and were now ready for a commitment. However, after another 2 years passed, David was again experiencing marital conflict and called to ask for a referral to a therapist in his area.

Example 4

Presentation

Norman, a 28-year-old scientist, asked for help to deal with the consequences of a divorce. At the same time, Norman had come close to being suspended from his job. He had misread his relationship with the head of the department, with whom he shared leftist political views, and had not considered the consequences of criticizing this man openly.

Norman's arrogance also led to the breakup of his marriage. Paula, whom he had met in school, was a rebel against her upper-class background and became involved in a series of causes. Again, Norman had to learn that political agreement does not predict interpersonal harmony. Paula found her husband to be unsupportive, unavailable, and unresponsive to feedback. She left him and later reconciled with her parents.

Norman had been raised in a family of ardent communists who had suffered persecution during the Cold War. Always involved in causes, his parents never made a steady living. Norman worked his way through college, which he saw as reflecting his solidarity with the underprivileged. He felt nothing but admiration for his family, with anger turned outward against any other form of authority.

Therapy

Identifying.   Working with Norman was difficult, largely because of his communication style. He would attempt to report encounters with people in detail, much as if he were a defendant on trial. His purpose was not to examine his own behavior but to prove that he was right, and even to give a political spin to the conflict. It was eventually possible to reach a point where Norman could acknowledge partial responsibility for his difficulties.

Observing.   Gradually Norman came to realize that his aggressiveness was defensive. In fact, he was exquisitely sensitive to interpersonal feedback. Moreover, he lacked the ability to soothe himself when stressful events occurred.

Experimenting.   Norman took steps to improve his work situation. He spent less time in the operating room, the setting where he had experienced the most trouble, and moved into research. There, he still had difficulty with collaboration but was able to control his environment more consistently.

In his interpersonal life, he mourned the loss of his wife and then moved into a new relationship with a nurse he met at the hospital. He described her to the therapist in glowing terms as having the supportive qualities he had missed in Paula.

Practicing.   Norman gradually became more comfortable with himself, although he still had something of a bad reputation in the laboratory. He left treatment after he obtained an academic position at a university and moved to another city, accompanied by his new partner.

Follow-Up Findings

Five years later, I heard from Norman again. He was quite successful in work, but was now going through a second divorce. Concerned about having sufficient access to his children, he asked me to testify at a civil hearing, with the idea was that I could support his case by confirming that he was a competent father. I pointed out, as gently as I could, that this was hardly the proper role for an ex-therapist. Moreover, if I were asked about why he was in treatment, I would have to explain his long-term difficulties getting along with people. Norman agreed that his case would go better without my testimony.

Working with Avoidant Personality Disorder

Patients with avoidant personality disorder (APD) are crippled by anxious traits. Psychotherapy has to help them to face and to master intense social anxiety. This behavioral aspect is a crucial element in treatment.

Formal studies of therapy for APD (Alden 1989; Stravynski et al. 1994) have demonstrated the effectiveness of social skills training, a behavioral method encouraging patients to overcome their anxiety and to learn new skills in dealing with people. We do not know the long-term outcome of these interventions, but the short-term results suggest the value of focused and pragmatic interventions.

In Chapter 5 I reviewed data suggesting that patients with Cluster B disorders are more likely to mature and improve in time than those whose pathology falls into Cluster C. My approach to APD accordingly sets conservative goals.

Some of these patients find a partner, possibly someone who accepts and enjoys being protective of them. In my experience, however, most never achieve intimacy. Therefore, it is particularly important for these patients to find other sources of satisfaction in life. They often benefit from working in a predictable environment and from having a few reliable friends. Although therapy should encourage patients to widen their options by facing fears, they usually seek out settings where rejection is unlikely.

Example 5

Presentation

Donna was an accountant in her early 30s who presented with long-term difficulties in establishing intimate relationships. She had a small circle of friends but had experienced only one love affair, a long-distance relationship. She was devoted to her work with clients. In this environment, she was able to relate helpfully in a context that was gratifying but unthreatening.

Donna had been unusually shy and awkward as a child. Moreover, she was raised in an impoverished family that provided little help with these difficulties. She had few friends and was painfully isolated in her adolescence. She responded by concentrating on her studies, at which she was successful. In this way, she could feel proud about having worked her way up in the world.

Therapy

Identifying.   Donna did not need to learn how to identify her maladaptive traits. She was all too well aware of them, as well as acutely conscious of her disabling social anxiety.

   Observing.   Donna focused on her reactions to new people and on attending social events. Both were to be avoided if possible. If not possible, these tasks required days of anxious preparation.

   Experimenting.   Therapy focused on strategies to overcome Donna's needs for withdrawal and safety. The emphasis was on gradual exposure to feared situations, as well as strategies for relaxation and distraction.

   Practicing.   In the course of therapy, Donna did not achieve intimacy. In her mind, this was an insurmountable hurdle. Yet she was able to establish a few stable friendships. Overall, she now spent less time at home.

Follow-Up Findings

A 20-year follow-up interview with Donna found her working at the same firm and still single. She had an intimate relationship with a divorced man, who, to her relief, had no interest in living with her. Once a year, she went on exotic travel with an old friend. Donna's life is not full, but she no longer feels anguished.

Summary

Therapy is a shared narrative. Yet too often, case histories are little more than fairy tales. They begin their stories with serious pathology but end happily—sometimes with the therapist receiving a slice of wedding cake!

   I am reminded of an encounter I had 25 years ago with the author of a well-known book about the psychotherapy of a troubled woman who had taken up a career as a high-class prostitute (Greenwald 1988). Although this was some years before I became formally involved in long-term follow-up research, I asked the therapist if he had heard from the patient recently. He sighed, then admitted to me that his "cured" patient was doing very badly indeed. Innocently, I asked him if he was planning to write up the outcome for a new edition of his book. Needless to say, he never did.

   None of the cases presented in this chapter has a classical happy ending. Even the best outcome (Example 1) is not that of an untroubled person but of someone who found a way around her troubles. The other patients obtained some benefit from treatment but continued to demonstrate fragility and difficulties over time. Given the chronicity of their problems, these patients often need to be seen at different stages of their life, each time with a somewhat different focus. Intermittent therapy may be the most appropriate and cost-effective prescription for patients with personality disorders.

Epilogue

A Program for Future Research

I end this book by noting what we do and do not know about the onset, course, and outcome of personality disorders. I then suggest directions that future research could take.

Most of the important questions about personality disorders have not been answered. As with other mental disorders, the precise links between temperament, traits, and disorder remain a mystery. Relationships between precursors and disorders are known to exist but are only statistical. We cannot predict with accuracy which children will go on to develop serious problems in adulthood. To address this issue, we need more longitudinal studies that follow children into adulthood. This type of research requires sophisticated designs and large samples.

Similarly, the relationship between personality disorders and their long-term outcome is replete with unanswered questions. Which patients can be expected to do well and why? For which patients are we best advised to invest our scarce resources? Again, we need longitudinal studies to answer these questions. Samples need to be large enough to take heterogeneity of outcome into account. Moreover, follow-up evaluation should not be limited to patients in therapy, who are not necessarily representative of this population.

Finally, we know surprisingly little about how to treat patients with personality disorders. The results of psychodynamic therapy have been somewhat disappointing. Hopeful new developments, such as dialectical behavior therapy, must be backed up with long-term follow-up data. Psychopharmacology must become less of a shotgun procedure and be more specifically targeted to produce clinically significant effects.

Researching all these questions will be expensive. Although it may take several more decades, such research could eventually produce some of the answers we are looking for. However, for research on personality disorders to be properly funded, the mental health community and the general public must first recognize the problem.

In the Introduction, I discussed why clinicians resist recognizing personality disorders. That situation is beginning to change. In recent years, there has been greater recognition within professional communities that these categories present major clinical problems. The National Institute of Mental Health (NIMH) has also recognized the issue, by funding a multisite study of the outcome for personality disordered patients. Moreover, the International Comorbidity Survey will be measuring the prevalence of two categories of personality disorders (instead of only one). A private foundation from Switzerland recently donated a large sum to research on the scientific understanding of borderline personality disorder.

Research must move in several directions. First and foremost, it must provide data necessary to support an etiological model of personality disorders. This book has presented some general ideas about that problem, but a definitive theory could look quite different. I suspect that, as with other mental disorders, genetics and the neurosciences will have to provide some of the answers. As long as we know so little about how the brain works, we cannot hope to understand phenomena as complex as personality disorders. We must find out how psychosocial factors interact with biological vulnerability to produce this form of pathology. It is also likely that advances in biological research will lead to a radically different classification of Axis II disorders.

Second, research can help us identify personality disorders at an earlier stage. Knowing who is most at risk will help us to target preventive interventions. My colleague Richard Tremblay, who has spent a lifetime studying antisocial behavior, has concluded that by the time antisocial children enter school, it may already be too late.

Third, research can provide us with a better description of the course and outcome of personality disorders. Here the NIMH Collaborative Study may play a crucial role. Whatever the vagaries of research funding, this is a project that should continue over the next 25 years. At the same time, because the cohorts in that study are all receiving therapy, it would also be helpful to conduct parallel research on the larger number of patients with personality disorders who do not seek treatment.

Finally, we have a desperate need for research on the treatment of personality disorders. Although I have been critical of the American Psychiatric Association guidelines for the treatment of borderline personality disorder, I hope that future editions of this document will have a much larger database to work with. I would also expect future editions to reach rather different conclusions from the "first pass" published in 2001.

The history of medicine shows that once we understand illness better, we eventually develop better treatments. I look forward to a time when clinicians will no longer wish to avoid patients with personality disorders. When we have more effective interventions, we will readily recognize these patients and welcome the opportunity to treat them.

References

Aarkrog T: Borderline adolescents 20 years later. Paper presented to the International Society for the Study of Personality Disorders, Cambridge, MA, September 1993

Achenbach TM, McConaughy SH: Empirically Based Assessment of Child and Adolescent Psychopathology: Practical Applications, 2nd Edition. Thousand Oaks, CA, Sage, 1997

Ad-Dab'bagh Y, Greenfield B: Multiple complex developmental disorder: the "multiple and complex" evolution of the "childhood borderline syndrome" construct. J Am Acad Child Adolesc Psychiatry 40:954–964, 2001

Adler G: Borderline Psychopathology and Its Treatment. New York, Jason Aronson, 1985

Alden L: Short-term structured treatment for avoidant personality disorder. J Consult Clin Psychol 57:756–764, 1989

Allen R: Discussion of paper by Meares and Stevenson. Aust N Z J Psychiatry 33:478–481, 1999

American Psychiatric Association: Diagnostic and Statistical Manual of Mental Disorders, 3rd Edition. Washington, DC, American Psychiatric Association, 1980

American Psychiatric Association: Diagnostic and Statistical Manual of Mental Disorders, 4th Edition. Washington, DC, American Psychiatric Association, 1994

American Psychiatric Association: Diagnostic and Statistical Manual of Mental Disorders, 4th Edition, Text Revision. Washington, DC, American Psychiatric Association, 2000

American Psychiatric Association: Guidelines for the Treatment of Borderline Personality Disorder. Am J Psychiatry 157(suppl):1–52, 2001

Apt C, Hurlbert DF: The sexual attitudes, behavior, and relationships of women with histrionic personality disorder. J Sex Marital Ther 20:125–133, 1994

Arboleda-Florez J, Holley HL: Antisocial burnout: an exploratory study. Bull Am Acad Psychiatry Law 19:173–183, 1991

Bandura A: Social Learning Theory. Englewood Cliffs, NJ, Prentice-Hall, 1977

Bardenstein KK, McGlashan TH: The natural history of a residentially treated borderline sample: gender differences. J Personal Disord 3:69–83, 1989

Barkley RA: Attention-Deficit Hyperactivity Disorder: A Handbook for Diagnosis and Treatment, 2nd Edition. New York, Guilford, 1998

Barr R: Malcolm X. San Diego, CA, Lucent Books, 1994

Bateman A, Fonagy P: Effectiveness of partial hospitalization in the treatment of borderline personality disorder: a randomized controlled trial. Am J Psychiatry 156:1563–1569, 1999

Bateman A, Fonagy P: Treatment of borderline personality disorder with psycho-analytically oriented partial hospitalization: an 18-month follow-up. Am J Psychiatry 158:36–42, 2001

Beck AT, Freeman A: Cognitive Therapy of Personality Disorders. New York, Guilford, 1990

Beers SR, De Bellis MD: Neuropsychological function in children with maltreatment-related posttraumatic stress disorder. Am J Psychiatry 159:483–486, 2002

Beilby W: Litigation in psychiatric practice. Presentation to the Canadian Psychiatric Association, Victoria, BC, October 2000

Bemporad JR, Ciccheti D: Borderline syndromes in childhood: criteria for diagnosis. Am J Psychiatry 139:596–601, 1982

Bender DS, Dolan RT, Skodol AE, et al: Treatment utilization by patients with personality disorders. Am J Psychiatry 158:295–302, 2001

Benjamin J, Patterson C, Greenberg BD, et al: Population and familial association between the D4 receptor gene and measures of novelty seeking. Nat Genet 12:81–84, 1996

Bergin AE, Garfield SL (eds): Handbook of Psychotherapy and Behavior Change. New York, Wiley, 1994

Bernstein DP, Cohen P, Velez CN, et al: Prevalence and stability of the DSM-III personality disorders in a community-based survey of adolescents. Am J Psychiatry 150:1237–1243, 1993

Berrios GE: European views on personality disorders: a conceptual history. Compr Psychiatry 34:14–30, 1993

Biederman J, Faraone S, Mick E, et al: Attention-deficit hyperactivity disorder and juvenile mania: an overlooked comorbidity? J Am Acad Child Adolesc Psychiatry 35:997–1008, 1996a

Bifulco A, Brown GW, Adler Z: Early sexual abuse and clinical depression in adult life. Br J Psychiatry 159:115–122, 1991

Bird G, Melville K: Families and Intimate Relationships. New York, McGraw-Hill, 1994

Black DW: Bad Boys, Bad Men: Confronting Antisocial Personality. New York, Oxford University Press, 1999

Black DW, Baumgard CH, Bell SE: A 16- to 45-year follow-up of 71 men with antisocial personality disorder. Compr Psychiatry 36:130–140, 1995

Black DW, Baumgard CH, Bell SE, Kao C: Death rates in 71 men with antisocial personality disorder: a comparison with general population mortality. Psychosomatics 37:131–136, 1996

Black DW, Monahan P, Baumgard CH, et al: Predictors of long-term outcome in 45 men with antisocial personality disorder. Ann Clin Psychiatry 19:211–217, 1997

Bland RC, Dyck RJ, Newman SC, et al: Attempted suicide in Edmonton, in Suicide in Canada. Edited by Leenaars AA, Wenckstern S, Sakinofsky I, et al. Toronto, ON, University of Toronto Press, 1998, pp 136–150

Bleuler E: Dementia Praecox of the Group of Schizophrenias. New York, International Universities Press, 1950

Bleuler M: The long-term course of the schizophrenic psychoses. Psychol Med 4:244–254, 1974

Block MJ, Westen D, Ludolph P, et al: Distinguishing female borderline adolescents from normal and other disturbed female adolescents. Psychiatry 54:89–103, 1991

Blumenthal SJ, Kupfer DJ (eds): Suicide Over the Life Cycle. Washington, DC, American Psychiatric Press, 1990

Bodlund O, Ekselius L, Lindstroem E: Personality traits and disorders among psychiatric outpatients and normal subjects on the basis of the SCID screen questionnaire. Nordic Journal of Psychiatry 47:425–433, 1993

Bongar BM (ed): Suicide: Guidelines for Assessment, Management, and Treatment. Washington, DC, American Psychological Association, 1992

Bongar B, Maris RW, Berman AL, et al: Outpatient standards of care and the suicidal patient, in Risk Management with Suicidal Patients. Edited by Bongar B, Berman AL, Maris RW, et al. New York, Guilford, 1998, pp 4–33

Bornstein RF: Dependent personality disorder in the DSM-IV and beyond. Clin Psychol Sci Pract 4:175–187, 1997

Bowlby J: Attachment. London, Hogarth Press, 1969

Bowman ML: Individual differences in posttraumatic distress: problems with the DSM-IV model. Can J Psychiatry 44:21–33, 1999

Braun-Scharm H: Suicidality and personality disorders in adolescence. Crisis: Journal of Crisis Intervention & Suicide 17:64–68, 1996

Brewin CR: Scientific status of recovered memories. Br J Psychiatry 169:131–134, 1996

Brieger P, Sommer S, Bloink F, et al: The relationship between five-factor personality measurements and ICD-10 personality disorder dimensions: results from a sample of 229 subjects. J Personal Disord 14:282–290, 2000

Browne A, Finkelhor D: Impact of child sexual abuse: a review of the literature. Psychol Bull 99:66–77, 1986

Buckley P, Karasu TB, Charles E: Psychotherapists view their personal therapy. Psychotherapy 18:299–305, 1981

Budman S, Denby A, Soldz S, et al: Time-limited group psychotherapy for patients with personality disorders: outcomes and drop-outs. Int J Group Psychother 46:357–377, 1996

Cadoret RJ, Yates WR, Troughton E, et al: Genetic environmental interaction in the genesis of aggressivity and conduct disorders. Arch Gen Psychiatry 52:916–924, 1995

Carpenter WT, Gunderson JG, Strauss JS: Considerations of the borderline syndrome: a longitudinal comparative study of borderline and schizophrenic patients, in Borderline Personality Disorders. Edited by Hartocollis P. New York, International Universities Press, 1977, pp 231–254

Carter JD, Joyce PR, Mulder RT, et al: Gender differences in the frequency of personality disorders in depressed outpatients. J Personal Disord 13:67–74, 1999

Casey PR: The epidemiology of personality disorder, in Personality Disorders: Diagnosis, Management, and Course, 2nd Edition. Edited by Tyrer P. Oxford, UK, Butterworth Heinemann, 2000, pp 71–80

Caspi A: The child is the father of the man: personality continuities from childhood to adulthood. J Pers Soc Psychol 78:158–172, 2000

Caspi A, Moffitt TE, Newman DL, et al: Behavioral observations at age three predict adult psychiatric disorders: longitudinal evidence from a birth cohort. Arch Gen Psychiatry 53:1033–1039, 1996

Chemtob CM, Hamada RS, Bauer GB, et al: Patient suicide: frequency and impact on psychiatrists. Am J Psychiatry 145:224–228, 1988a

Chemtob CM, Hamada RS, Bauer GB, et al: Patient suicide: frequency and impact on psychiatrists. Professional Psychology: Research and Practice 19:416–420, 1988b

Chess S, Thomas A: Origins and Evolution of Behavior Disorders: From Infancy to Adult Life. New York, Brunner/Mazel, 1984

Chessick R: Intensive psychotherapy of the borderline patient. New York, Jason Aronson, 1985

Cheung P: Adult psychiatric epidemiology in China in the 1980's. Culture, Medicine, Psychiatry 15:479–496, 1991

Childs B: Genetics, evolution, and age at onset of disease, in Childhood Onset of Adult Psychopathology: Clinical and Research Advances. Edited by Rapaport J. Washington, DC, American Psychiatric Press, 2000, pp 27–40

Ciompi L: The natural history of schizophrenia in the long term. Br J Psychiatry 136:413–420, 1980

Clark LA, Livesley WJ: Two approaches to identifying the dimensions of personality disorder: convergence on the five-factor model, in Personality Disorders and the Five-Factor Model of Personality, 2nd Edition. Edited by Costa PJ, Widiger TA. Washington, DC, American Psychological Association, 2002, pp 161–176

Cleckley H: The Mask of Sanity, 4th Edition. St. Louis, MO, Mosby, 1964

Cloninger CR: A systematic method for clinical description and classification of personality variants. Arch Gen Psychiatry 44:579–588, 1987

Cloninger CR, Sigvardsson S, Bohman M, et al: Predisposition to petty criminality in Swedish adoptees. Arch Gen Psychiatry 39:1242–1247, 1982

Cloninger CR, Svrakic DM, Pryzbeck TR: A psychobiological model of temperament and character. Arch Gen Psychiatry 50:975–990, 1993

Coccaro EF: Clinical outcome of psychopharmacologic treatment of borderline and schizotypal personality disordered subjects. J Clin Psychiatry 59(suppl 1):30–35, 1998

Coccaro EF, Kavoussi RJ: Fluoxetine and impulsive aggressive behavior in personality-disordered subjects. Arch Gen Psychiatry 54:1081–1088, 1997

Coccaro EF, Siever LJ, Klar HM, et al: Serotonergic studies in patients with affective and personality disorders. Arch Gen Psychiatry 46:587–599, 1989

Cohen DJ, Paul R, Volkmar F: Issues in the classification of pervasive developmental disorders and associated conditions, in Handbook of Autism and Pervasive Developmental Disorders. Edited by Cohen DJ, Donnelean AM. New York, Wiley, 1987, pp 20–39

Compton WM 3rd, Helzer JE, Hwu HG, et al: New methods in cross-cultural psychiatry: psychiatric illness in Taiwan and the United States. Am J Psychiatry 148:1697–1704, 1991

Conrod PJ, Pihl RO, Stewart SH, et al: Validation of a system of classifying female substance abusers on the basis of personality and motivational risk factors for substance abuse. Psychol Addict Behav 14:243–256, 2000

Cornelius JR, Soloff PH, Perel JM, et al: Continuation pharmacotherapy of borderline personality disorder with haloperidol and phenelzine. Am J Psychiatry 150:1843–1848, 1993

Costa PT, McCrae RR: From catalog to Murray's needs and the five factor model. J Pers Soc Psychol 55:258–265, 1988

Costa PT, Widiger TA (eds): Personality Disorders and the Five-Factor Model of Personality. Washington, DC, American Psychological Association, 1994

Costa PT, Widiger TA (eds): Personality Disorders and the Five-Factor Model of Personality, 2nd Edition. Washington, DC, American Psychological Association, 2001

Courtless T: Commitment of mentally disordered criminal offenders in the state of Maryland: future dangerousness versus treatment amenability. Journal of Forensic Psychiatry 8:417–433, 1997

Cowdry RW, Gardner DL: Pharmacotherapy of borderline personality disorder: alprazolam, carbamazepine, trifluoperazine, and tranylcypromine. Arch Gen Psychiatry 45:111–119, 1988

Crawford TN, Cohen P, Brook JS: Dramatic-erratic personality disorder symptoms, I: continuity from early adolescence to adulthood. J Pers Disorders 15:319–335, 2001a

Crawford TN, Cohen P, Brook JS: Dramatic-erratic personality disorder symptoms, II: developmental pathways from early adolescence to adulthood. J Pers Disorders 15:336–350, 2001b

Crow S, Praus B, Thuras P: Mortality from eating disorders: a 5- to 10-year record linkage study. Int J Eating Disord 26:97–101, 1999

Dawson D, MacMillan HL: Relationship Management of the Borderline Patient: From Understanding to Treatment. New York, Brunner/Mazel, 1993

Demopoulos C, Fava M, McLean NE, et al: Hypochondriacal concerns in depressed outpatients. Psychosom Med 58:314–320, 1996

Derogatis L: SCL-90: administration, scoring, and procedures manual norms. Minneapolis, MN, National Computer Systems, 1994 deVries MW: Kids in context: temperament in cross-cultural perspective, in Prevention and Early Intervention: Individual Differences as Risk Factors for the Mental Health of Children. Edited by Carey WB, McDevitt S, Conway S. Philadelphia, PA, Brunner/Mazel, 1994, pp 126–139

Dicks HV: Marital Tensions. New York, Basic Books, 1967

Dolan B, Coid J: Psychopathic and antisocial personality disorders: treatment and research issues. London, Gaskell/Royal College of Psychiatrists, 1993

Drake RE, Gates C: Suicide among schizophrenics: who is at risk? J Nerv Ment Dis 172:613–617, 1984

Dulit RA, Fyer MR, Miller FT, et al: Gender differences in sexual preference and substance abuse of inpatients with borderline personality disorder. J Personal Disord 7:182–185, 1993

Elkin I, Shea T, Watkins JT, et al: National Institute of Mental Health Treatment of Depression Collaborative Research Program: general effectiveness of treatments. Arch Gen Psychiatry 46:971–982, 1989

Endicott J, Spitzer RL, Fleiss JL, et al: The global assessment scale: a procedure for measuring overall severity of psychiatric disorder. Arch Gen Psychiatry 33:766–772, 1976

Erikson E: Childhood and Society. New York, Norton, 1950

Erlenmeyer-Kimling L, Rock D, Roberts SA, et al: Attention, memory, and motor skills as childhood predictors of schizophrenia-related psychoses: the New York High-Risk Project. Am J Psychiatry 157:1416–1422, 2000

Eysenck H: The effects of psychotherapy: an evaluation. J Consult Psychol 16:319–324, 1952

Eysenck HJ: Crime and Personality. London, Paladin, 1977

Ezpeleta L, Keeler G, Alaatin E, et al: Epidemiology of psychiatric disability in childhood and adolescence. J Child Psychol Psychiatry 42:901–914, 2001

Falconer DS: Introduction to Quantitative Genetics. Essex, UK, Longman, 1989

Fava M: Psychopharmacologic treatment of pathologic aggression. Psychiatr Clin North Am 20:427–451, 1997

Feldman RB, Zelkowitz P, Weiss M, et al: A comparison of the families of borderline personality disorder mothers and the families of other personality disorder mothers. Compr Psychiatry 36:157–163, 1995

Fine MA, Sansone RA: Dilemmas in the management of suicidal behavior in individuals with borderline personality disorder. Am J Psychother 44:160–171, 1990

Flavin DK, Franklin JE Jr, Frances RJ: Substance abuse and suicidal behavior, in Suicide over the Life Cycle: Risk Factors, Assessment, and Treatment of Suicidal Patients. Edited by Blumenthal SJ, Kupfer DJ. Washington, DC, American Psychiatric Press, 1990, pp 177–204

Fombonne E, Worstear G, Cooper V, et al: The Maudsley long-term follow-up of depressed adolescents. Br J Psychiatry 179:210–217, 2001

Frank E (ed): Gender and Its Effects on Psychopathology. Washington, DC, American Psychiatric Press, 2000

Frank E, Young E: Pubertal changes and adolescent challenges: why do rates of depression rise precipitously for girls between ages 10 and 15 years? in Gender and Its Effects on Psychopathology. Edited by Frank E. Washington, DC, American Psychiatric Press, 2000, pp 85–102

Frank JD, Frank JB: Persuasion and Healing, 3rd Edition. Baltimore, MD, Johns Hopkins University Press, 1991

Freud S: Analysis terminable and interminable, in The Standard Edition of the Psychological Works of Sigmund Freud, Vol XXIII. Edited by Strachey J. London, Hogarth, 1937 (reprinted 1964), pp 216–254

Gabbard GO, Coyne L: Predictors of response of antisocial patients to hospital treatment. Hosp Community Psychiatry 38:1181–1185, 1987

Garnet KE, Levy KN, Mattanana BA, et al: Borderline personality disorder in adolescents: ubiquitous or specific. Am J Psychiatry 151:1380–1382, 1994

Goldberg D: Plato versus Aristotle: categorical and dimensional models for common mental disorders. Compr Psychiatry 41(suppl):8–13, 2000

Goldman SJ, D'Angelo EJ, DeMaso DR, et al: Physical and sexual abuse histories among children with borderline personality disorder. Am J Psychiatry 149:1723–1726, 1992

Goldman SJ, D'Angelo EJ, DeMaso DR: Psychopathology in the families of children and adolescents with borderline personality disorder. Am J Psychiatry 150:1832–1835, 1993

Goldstein RB, Black DW, Nasrallah A, et al: The prediction of suicide. Arch Gen Psychiatry 48:418–422, 1991

Goodwin DW, Warnock JK: Alcoholism: a family disease, in Clinical Textbook of Addictive Disorders. Edited by Frances RJ, Miller SI. New York, Guilford, 1991, pp 485–500

Gottesman I: Schizophrenia Genesis. New York, Freeman, 1991

Gottman JM, Levenson RW: The timing of divorce: predicting when a couple will divorce over a 14-year period. J Marriage Family 62:737–745, 2000

Greenman DA, Gunderson JG, Cane M, et al: An examination of the borderline diagnosis in children. Am J Psychiatry 143:998–1002, 1986

Greenwald H: The Call Girl. New York, Libra, 1988

Grilo CM, McGlashan TH, Skodol AE: Stability and course of personality disorders. Psychiatr Q 71:291–307, 2000

Grilo CM, Becker DF, Edell WS, et al: Stability and change of DSM-III-R personality disorder dimensions in adolescents followed up 2 years after psychiatric hospitalization. Compr Psychiatry 42:364–368, 2001

Gross R, Olfson M, Gameroff M, et al: Borderline personality disorder in primary care. Arch Intern Med 162:53–60, 2002

Guilé JM: Narcissistic personality disorder characteristics in children. Presentation to the Personality Disorders Research Network, McGill University, Montreal, Quebec, Canada, April 2000

Gunderson JG: Borderline Personality Disorder: A Clinical Guide. Washington, DC, American Psychiatric Press, 2001

Gunderson JG, Phillips KA: A current view of the interface between borderline personality disorder and depression. Am J Psychiatry 148:967–975, 1991

Gunderson JG, Ronningstam E: Differentiating narcissistic and antisocial personality disorders. J Personal Disord 15:103–109, 2001

Gunderson JG, Frank AF, Ronningstam EF, et al: Early discontinuance of borderline patients from psychotherapy. J Nerv Ment Dis 177:38–42, 1989

Gunderson JG, Ronningstam E, Bodkin A: The diagnostic interview for narcissistic patients. Arch Gen Psychiatry 47:676–680, 1990

Gunderson JG, Shea MT, Skodol AE, et al: The Collaborative Longitudinal Personality Disorders Study: development, aims, design, and sample characteristics. J Personal Disord 14:300–315, 2000

Gurvits IG, Koenigsberg HW, Siever LJ: Neurotransmitter dysfunction in patients with borderline personality disorder. Psychiatr Clin North Am 23:27–40, 2000

Gutheil TG: Suicide and suit: liability after self-destruction, in Suicide and Clinical Practice. Edited by Jacobs D. Washington, DC, American Psychiatric Press, 1992, pp 147–167

Guzder J, Paris J, Zelkowitz P, et al: Risk factors for borderline pathology in children. J Am Acad Child Adolesc Psychiatry 35:26–33, 1996

Guzder J, Paris J, Zelkowitz P, et al: Psychological risk factors for borderline pathology in school-aged children. J Am Acad Child Adolesc Psychiatry 38:206–212, 1999

Guze JB, Robins E: Suicide and primary affective disorders. Br J Psychiatry 117:437–438, 1970

Hamburger ME, Lilienfeld SO, Hogben M: Psychopathy, gender, and gender roles: implications for antisocial and histrionic personality disorders. J Personal Disord 10:41–55, 1996

Harding CM, Keller H: Long-term outcome of social functioning, in Handbook of Social Functioning in Schizophrenia. Edited by Mueser KT, Tarrier N. Boston, MA, Allyn and Bacon, 1998, pp 134–148

Harding CM, Brooks GW, Ashikaga T, et al: Vermont Longitudinal Study of persons with severe mental illness. Am J Psychiatry 143:727–735, 1987

Harpur TJ, Hart SD, Hare RD: Personality of the psychopath, in Personality Disorders and the Five-Factor Model. Edited by Costa PT, Widiger TA. Washington, DC, American Psychological Association, 1994, pp 149–174

Harrington R, Rutter M, Fombonne E: Developmental pathways in depression: multiple meanings, antecedents, and endpoints. Dev Psychopathol 8:601–616, 1996

Harrison G, Hopper T, Craig E, et al: Recovery from psychotic illness: a 15- and 25-year international follow-up study. Br J Psychiatry 178:506–517, 2001

Hart SD, Hare RD: Psychopathy and the big 5: correlations between observers' ratings of normal and pathological personality. J Personal Disord 8:32–40, 1994

Head SB, Baker JD, Williamson DA: Family environment characteristics and dependent personality disorder. J Personal Disord 5:256–263, 1991

Hechtman L (ed): Do They Grow Out of It? Washington, DC, American Psychiatric Press, 1996

Helzer JE, Canino GJ (eds): Alcoholism in North America, Europe, and Asia. New York, Oxford University Press, 1992

Herrell R, Goldberg J, True WR, et al: Sexual orientation and suicidality: a co-twin control study in adult men. Arch Gen Psychiatry 56:867–874, 1999

Hoge SK, Appelbaum PS, Greer A: An empirical comparison of the stone and dangerousness criteria for civil commitment. Am J Psychiatry 146:170–175, 1989

Høglend P: Personality disorders and long-term outcome after brief dynamic psychotherapy. J Personal Disord 7:168–181, 1993

Hollander E, Allen A, Lopez RP, et al: A preliminary double-blind, placebo-controlled trial of divalproex sodium in borderline personality disorder. J Clin Psychiatry 62:199–203, 2001

Horwitz L: Clinical Prediction in Psychotherapy. New York, Jason Aronson, 1974

Hser Y-I, Hoffman V, Grella CE, et al: A 33-year follow-up of narcotics addicts. Arch Gen Psychiatry 58:503–508, 2001

Huber G, Gross G, Schuttler R: A long-term follow-up study of schizophrenia: psychiatric course of illness and prognosis. Acta Psychiatr Scand 50:49–57, 1975

Hughes R: The Fatal Shore. New York, Vintage, 1988

Hull JW, Yeomans F, Clarkin J, et al: Factors associated with multiple hospitalizations of patients with borderline personality disorder. Psychiatr Serv 47:638–641, 1996

Hwu HG, Yeh EK, Change LY: Prevalence of psychiatric disorders in Taiwan defined by the Chinese Diagnostic Interview Schedule. Acta Psychiatr Scand 79:136–147, 1989

Inkeles A, Smith DH: Becoming Modern: Individual Change in Six Developing Countries. Cambridge, MA, Harvard University Press, 1974

Isacsson G, Bergman U, Rich CL: Epidemiological data suggest antidepressants reduce suicide risk among depressives. J Affect Disord 41:1–8, 1996

Jacobsen N, Gurman A (eds): Clinical Handbook of Couple Therapy. New York, Guilford, 1995

James A, Berelowitz M, Vereker M: Borderline personality disorder: study in adolescence. Eur Child Adolesc Psychiatry 5:11–17, 1996

Jang KL, Livesley WJ, Vernon PA, et al: Heritability of personality traits: a twin study. Acta Psychiatr Scand 94:438–444, 1996

Jang KL, Paris J, Zweig-Frank H, et al: Twin study of dissociative experience. J Nerv Ment Dis 186:345–351, 1998

Jennings C, Barraclough BM, Moss JR: Have the Samaritans lowered the suicide rate? A controlled study. Psychol Med 8:413–422, 1978

Johnson BA, Brent DA, Connolly J, et al: Familial aggregation of adolescent personality disorders. J Am Acad Child Adolesc Psychiatry 34:798–804, 1995

Johnson JG, Cohen P, Skodol AE, et al: Personality disorders in adolescence and risk of major mental disorders and suicidality during adulthood. Arch Gen Psychiatry 56:805–811, 1999

Johnson JJ, Cohen P, Brown J, et al: Childhood maltreatment increases risk for personality disorders during early adulthood. Arch Gen Psychiatry 56:600–606, 1999

Jones M: The Therapeutic Community. New York, Basic Books, 1953

Kagan J: Unstable Ideas: Temperament, Cognition and Self. Cambridge, MA, Harvard University Press, 1989

Kagan J: Galen's Prophecy. New York, Basic Books, 1994

Kagan J, Zentner M: Early childhood predictors of adult psychopathology. Harv Rev Psychiatry 3:341–350, 1996

Kasen S, Cohen P, Skodol AE, et al: Influence of child and adolescent psychiatric disorders on young adult personality disorder. Am J Psychiatry 156:1529–1535, 1999

Kasen S, Cohen P, Skodol AE, et al: Childhood Depression and Adult Personality Disorder: Alternative Pathways of Continuity. Arch Gen Psychiatry 58:231–236, 2001

Kaufman J, Martin A, King RA, et al: Are child-, adolescent-, and adult-onset depression one and the same disorder? Biol Psychiatry 49:980–1001, 2001

Kavoussi RJ, Coccaro EF: Divalproex sodium for impulsive aggressive behavior in patients with personality disorder. J Clin Psychiatry 59:676–680, 1998

Kazdin AE: Treatment of conduct disorders, in Conduct Disorders in Childhood and Adolescence. Edited by Hill J, Maughan B. New York, Cambridge University Press, 2001, pp 408–448

Keel PK, Mitchell JE, Miller KB, et al: Long-term outcome of bulimia nervosa. Arch Gen Psychiatry 56:63–69, 1999

Kelley JT: Psychiatric Malpractice: Stories of Patients, Psychiatrists, and the Law. New Brunswick, NJ, Rutgers University Press, 1996

Kendler KS: Genetic epidemiology in psychiatry: taking both genes and environment seriously. Arch Gen Psychiatry 52:895–899, 1995

Kendler KS, Gardner CO: Boundaries of major depression: an evaluation of DSM-IV criteria. Am J Psychiatry 155:172–177, 1998

Kendler KS, Gruenberg AM, Strauss JJ: An independent analysis of the Copenhagen sample of the Danish Adoption Study of Schizophrenia. II: the relationship between schizotypal personality disorder and schizophrenia. Arch Gen Psychiatry 38:983–984, 1981

Kendler KS, McGuire MM, Gruenberg AM, et al: The Roscommon family study, I: methods, diagnosis of probands, and risk of schizophrenia in relatives. Arch Gen Psychiatry 50:527–540, 1993

Kernberg OF: Borderline Conditions and Pathological Narcissism. New York, Jason Aronson, 1976

Kernberg OF: Severe Personality Disorders. New York, Basic Books, 1987

Kernberg P: Personality disorders, in American Academy of Child and Adolescent Psychiatry Textbook of Child and Adolescent Psychiatry. Edited by Weiner J. Washington, DC, American Psychiatric Press, 1991, pp 515–533

Kernberg OF, Coyne L, Appelbaum A, et al: Final report of the Menninger Psychotherapy Research Project. Bull Menninger Clin 36:1–275, 1972

Kernberg PF, Weiner AS, Bardenstein KK: Personality Disorders in Children and Adolescents. New York, Basic Books, 2000

Keshavan MS, Anderson S, Pettegrew JW: Is schizophrenia due to excessive synaptic pruning in the prefrontal cortex? The Feinberg hypothesis revisited. J Psychiatr Res 28:239–265, 1994

Kessing LV, Andersen PK, Mortensen PB: Predictors of recurrence in affective disorder: a case register study. J Affect Disord 49:101–108, 1998

Kessler RC, McGonagle KA, Nelson CB, et al: Lifetime and 12-month prevalence of DSM-III-R psychiatric disorders in the United States. Arch Gen Psychiatry 51:8–19, 1994

Kestenbaum CJ: The borderline child at risk for major psychiatric disorder in adult life, in The Borderline Child. Edited by Robson KR. New York, McGraw Hill, 1983, pp 49–82

Kish GB: CPI correlates of stimulus-seeking in male alcoholics. J Clin Psychol 27:251–253, 1971

Kjelsberg E, Eikeseth PH, Dahl AA: Suicide in borderline patients—predictive factors. Acta Psychiatr Scand 84:283–287, 1991

Kjelsberg E, Neegaard E, Dahl AA: Suicide in adolescent psychiatric inpatients: incidence and predictive factors. Acta Psychiatr Scand 89:235–241, 1994

Klerman GL: The psychiatric patient's right to effective treatment: Implications of Osheroff v. Chestnut Lodge. Am J Psychiatry 147:409–418, 1990

Koenig HG: Religion and medicine II: Religion, mental health, and related behaviors. Int J Psychiatr Med 31:97–109, 2001

Koenigsberg HW, Harvey PD, Mitropoulou V, et al: Characterizing Affective Instability in Borderline Personality Disorder. Am J Psychiatry 159:784–788, 2002

Koerner K, Linehan MM: Research on dialectical behavior therapy for patients with borderline personality disorder. Psychiatr Clin North Am 23:151–167, 2002

Kohut H: The Analysis of the Self. New York, International Universities Press, 1970

Kohut H: The Restoration of the Self. New York, International Universities Press, 1977

Koons CR, Robins CJ, Bishop GK, et al: Efficacy of dialectical behavior therapy with borderline women veterans: a randomized controlled trial. Behav Ther 32:371–390, 2001

Kopta SM, Howard KI, Lowry JL, et al: Patterns of symptomatic recovery in psychotherapy. J Consult Clin Psychol 62:1009–1016, 1994

Kraepelin E: Dementia Praecox and Paraphrenia. Translated by Barclay M. Edinburgh, Scotland, Livingstone, 1919

Kroll J: The Challenge of the Borderline Patient. New York, Norton, 1988

Kroll J: PTSD/Borderlines in Therapy. New York, Norton, 1993

Krueger RF: The structure of common mental disorders. Arch Gen Psychiatry 56:921–926, 1999

Kullgren G: Factors associated with completed suicide in borderline personality disorder. J Nerv Ment Dis 176:40–44, 1988

Kumra S, Jacobsen LK, Lenane M, et al: "Multidimensionally impaired disorder": is it a variant of very early onset schizophrenia? J Am Acad Child Adolesc Psychiatry 37:91–99, 1998

Laub JH, Vaillant GE: Delinquency and mortality: A 50-year follow-up study of 1,000 delinquent and nondelinquent boys. Am J Psychiatry 157:96–102, 2000

Lee KC, Kovac YS, Rhee H: The national epidemiological study of mental disorders in Korea. J Korean Med Sci 2:19–34, 1987

Lee RB: Politics, sexual and non-sexual in an egalitarian society. Social Science Information 17:871–895, 1978

Leibenluft E, Gardner DL, Cowdry RW: The inner experience of the borderline self-mutilator. J Personal Disord l:317–324, 1987

Lenzenweger MF, Loranger AW, Korfine L, et al: Detecting personality disorders in a nonclinical population: application of a 2-stage for case identification. Arch Gen Psychiatry 54:345–351, 1997

Lerner D: The Passing of Traditional Society, New York, Free Press, 1958

Lesage AD, Boyer R, Grunberg F, et al: Suicide and mental disorders: a case control study of young men. Am J Psychiatry 151:1063–1068, 1994

Lesch KP, Bengel D, Heils A, et al: Association of anxiety-related traits with a polymorphism in the serotonin transporter gene regulatory region. Science 274:1527–1531, 1996

Leventhal EA: Biology of aging, in Comprehensive Review of Geriatric Psychiatry, 2nd Edition. Edited by Sadavoy J, Lazarus L. Washington, DC, American Psychiatric Press, 1996, pp 81–112

Lewis L, Appleby L: Personality disorder: the patients psychiatrists dislike. Br J Psychiatry 153:44–49, 1988

Leyton M, Okazawa H, Diksic M, et al: Brain regional rate alpha-[^{11}C]methyl-L-tryptophan trapping in impulsive subjects with borderline personality disorder. Am J Psychiatry 158:775–782, 2001

Lincoln AJ, Bloom D, Katz M, et al: Neuropsychological and neurophysiological indices of auditory processing impairment in children with multiple complex developmental disorder. J Am Acad Child Adolesc Psychiatry 37:100–112, 1998

Linehan MM: Dialectical Behavioral Therapy of Borderline Personality Disorder. New York, Guilford, 1993

Linehan MM: Update on DBT. Paper presented to the International Society for the Study of Personality Disorders, Geneva, Switzerland, September 1999

Linehan MM, Armstrong HE, Suarez A, et al: Cognitive behavioral treatment of chronically parasuicidal borderline patients. Arch Gen Psychiatry 48:1060–1064, 1991

Linehan MM, Heard HL, Armstrong HE: Naturalistic follow-up of a behavioral treatment for chronically parasuicidal borderline patients. Arch Gen Psychiatry 50:971–974, 1993

Links PS, Steiner B, Huxley G: The occurrence of borderline personality disorder in the families of borderline patients. J Personal Disord 2:14–20, 1988

Links PS, Steiner M, Boiago I, et al: Lithium therapy for borderline patients: preliminary findings. J Personal Disord 4:173–181, 1990

Links PS, Heslegrave RJ, Mitton JE, et al: Borderline personality disorder and substance abuse: consequences of comorbidity. Can J Psychiatry 40:9–14, 1995

Links PS, Heslegrave R, van Reekum R: Prospective follow-up study of borderline personality disorder: prognosis, prediction of outcome, and Axis II comorbidity. Can J Psychiatry 43:265–270, 1998

Liskow BI, Powell BJ, Penick EC, et al: Mortality in male alcoholics after ten to fourteen years. J Stud Alcohol 61:853–61, 2000

Livesley WJ: The Practical Management of Personality Disorder. New York, Guilford (in press)

Livesley WJ, Jang KL, Vernon PA: Phenotypic and genetic structure of traits delineating personality disorder. Arch Gen Psychiatry 55:941–948, 1998

Lofgren DP, Bemporad J, King J, et al: A prospective follow-up study of so-called borderline children. Am J Psychiatry 148:1541–1545, 1991

Looper K, Paris J: What are the dimensions underlying Cluster B personality disorders? Compr Psychiatry 41:432–437, 2000

Loranger AW: Dependent personality disorder: age, sex, and Axis I comorbidity. J Nerv Ment Dis 184:17–21, 1996

Luborsky L: Clinicians' judgment of mental health. Arch Gen Psychiatry 9:407–417, 1963

Ludolph PS, Westen D, Misle B: The borderline diagnosis in adolescents: symptoms and developmental history. Am J Psychiatry 147:470–476, 1990

Luhrmann TM: Of two minds: the growing disorder in American psychiatry. New York, Knopf, 2000

Lykken D: The Antisocial Personalities. Hillside, NJ, Erlbaum, 1995

Maccoby EE, Jacklin CN: The Psychology of Sex Differences. Stanford, CA, Stanford University Press, 1974

Maddocks PD: A five year follow-up of untreated psychopaths. Br J Psychiatry 116:511–515, 1970

Malan D: Individual Psychotherapy and the Science of Psychodynamics. Boston, MA, Butterworths, 1979

Maltsberger JT: Calculated risk in the treatment of intractably suicidal patients. Psychiatry 57:199–212, 1994

Mann JJ: The neurobiology of suicide. Nat Med 4:25–30, 1998

Maris RW: Pathways to Suicide. Baltimore, MD, Johns Hopkins University Press, 1981

Maris RW: Suicide. Lancet 360:319–326, 2002

Markowitz PJ: Pharmacotherapy of impulsivity, aggression, and related disorders, in Impulsivity and Aggression. Edited by Hollander E, Stein DJ. New York, John Wiley, 1995, pp 263–286

Masse LC, Tremblay RE: Behavior of boys in kindergarten and the onset of substance use during adolescence. Arch Gen Psychiatry 54:62–68, 1997

Masters RD, McGuire MT: The Neurotransmitter Revolution: Serotonin, Social Behavior, and the Law. Carbondale, IL, South Illinois Press, 1994

Mattanah BA, Becker DF, Levy KN, et al: Diagnostic stability in adolescents followed up 2 years after hospitalization. Am J Psychiatry 152:889–894, 1995

Mattia JL, Zimmerman M: Epidemiology, in Handbook of Personality Disorders. Edited by Livesley WJ. New York, Guilford, 2001, pp 107–123

Maughan B, Rutter M: Retrospective reporting of childhood adversity. J Personal Disord 11:4–18, 1997

Mavissakalian MR, Hamann MS, Abou Haidar S, et al: DSM-III personality disorders in generalized anxiety, panic/agoraphobia, and obsessive-compulsive disorders. Compr Psychiatry 34:243–248, 1993

McCrae RR, Costa PT: A five-factor theory of personality, in Handbook of Personality: Theory and Research, 2nd Edition. Edited by Pervin LA, John OP. New York, Guilford, 1999, pp 139–153

McDavid JD, Pilkonis PA: The stability of personality disorder diagnoses. J Personal Disord 10:1–15, 1996

McGlashan TH: The prediction of outcome in borderline personality disorder, in The Borderline: Current Empirical Research. Edited by McGlashan TH. Washington, DC, American Psychiatric Press, 1985, pp 61–98

McGlashan TH: The Chestnut Lodge follow-up study, III: long-term outcome of borderline personalities. Arch Gen Psychiatry 43:2–30, 1986a

McGlashan TH: The Chestnut Lodge follow-up study, VI: schizotypal personality disorder. Arch Gen Psychiatry 43:329–334, 1986b

McGlashan TH: The schizophrenia spectrum concept: the Chestnut Lodge follow-up study. Schizophr Res 1:193–200, 1991

McGlashan TH: Implications of outcome research for the treatment of borderline personality disorder, in Borderline Personality Disorder: Etiology and Treatment. Edited by Paris J. Washington, DC, American Psychiatric Press, 1993, pp 235–260

McGlashan TH: The borderline personality disorder practice guidelines: the good, the bad, and the realistic. J Personal Disord 16:119–121, 2002

McGuffin P, Gottesman I: Genetic influences on normal and abnormal development, in Child and Adolescent Psychiatry: Modern Approaches. Edited by Rutter M, Hersov L. Oxford, UK, Blackwell, 1985, pp 17–33

McGuffin P, Katz J, Watkins S, et al: A hospital-based twin register of the heritability of DSM-IV unipolar depression. Arch Gen Psychiatry 53:129–136, 1996

McNeil TF, Cantor-Graae E, Weinberger DR: Relationship of obstetric complications and differences in size of brain structures in monozygotic twin pairs discordant for schizophrenia. Am J Psychiatry 157:203–212, 2000

Meares R, Stevenson J, Comerford A: Psychotherapy with borderline patients, I: a comparison between treated and untreated cohorts. Austr N Z J Psychiatry 33:467–472, 1999

Mednick SA, Cudeck R, Griffith JJ, et al: The Danish High-Risk Project: recent methods and findings, in Children at Risk for Schizophrenia: A Longitudinal Perspective. Edited by Watt NF, Anthony EJ. New York, Cambridge University Press, 1984, pp 21–42

Meehl PE: Toward an integrated theory of schizotaxa, schizotypy, and schizophrenia. J Personal Disord 4:1–99, 1990

Michaels S: The prevalence of homosexuality in the United States, in Textbook of Homosexuality and Mental Health. Edited by Cabaj RJ, Stein TS. Washington, DC, American Psychiatric Press, 1996, pp 43–63

Millon T: Borderline personality disorder: a psychosocial epidemic, in Borderline Personality Disorder: Etiology and Treatment. Edited by Paris J. Washington, DC, American Psychiatric Press, 1993, pp 197–210

Mirsky AF, Bieliauskas LA, French LM, et al: A 39-year follow-up of the Genain quadruplets. Schizophr Bull 26:699–708, 2000

Moeller FG, Barratt ES, Dougherty DM, et al: Psychiatric aspects of impulsivity. Am J Psychiatry 158:1783–1793, 2001

Moffitt TE: "Life-course persistent" and "adolescence-limited" antisocial behavior: a developmental taxonomy. Psychol Rev 100:674–701, 1993

Moffitt TE, Caspi A, Rutter MM, Silva PA: Sex differences in antisocial behavior. New York, Cambridge University Press, 2001

Monroe SM, Simons AD: Diathesis-stress theories in the context of life stress research. Psychol Bull 110:406–425, 1991

Monsen JT, Odland T, Faugli A, et al: Personality disorders: changes and stability after intensive psychotherapy focusing on affect consciousness. Psychother Res 5:33–48, 1995

Moos RH: Conceptual and empirical approaches to developing family-based assessment procedures: resolving the case of the Family Environment Scale. Family Process 29:199–208, 1990

Munroe-Blum H: Group treatment of borderline personality disorder, in Borderline Personality Disorder: Clinical and Empirical Perspectives. Edited by Clarkin JF, Marziali E, Munroe-Blum H. New York, Guilford, 1992, pp 288–299

Munroe-Blum H, Marziali E: A controlled trial of short-term group treatment for borderline personality disorder. J Personal Disord 9:190–198, 1995

Murphy HBM: Comparative Psychiatry. New York, Springer, 1982

Murray RM, Van Os J: Predictors of outcome in schizophrenia. J Clin Psychopharmacol 18(suppl 1):2S–4S, 1998

Nace EP, Davis CW: Treatment outcome in substance-abusing patients with a personality disorder. Am J Addict 2:26–33, 1993

Najavits LM, Gunderson JG: Better than expected: improvements in borderline personality disorder in a 3-year prospective outcome study. Compr Psychiatry 36:296–302, 1995

Narrow WE, Rae DS, Robins LN, et al: Revised prevalence estimates of mental disorders in the United States. Arch Gen Psychiatry 59:115–123, 2002

Nasar S: A Beautiful Mind. New York, Simon and Schuster, 1998

Nesse R, Williams GC: Why We Get Sick. New York, Random House, 1994

Nestadt G, Romanovski AJ, Chahal R, et al: An epidemiological study of histrionic personality disorder. Psychol Med 20:413–422, 1990

Newman SC, Bland RC: Incidence of mental disorders in Edmonton: estimates of rates and methodological issues. J Psychiatr Res 32:273–282, 1998

Nicolson R, Lenane M, Brookner F, et al: Children and adolescents with psychotic disorder not otherwise specified: a 2- to 8-year follow-up study. J Am Acad Child Adolesc Psychiatry 42:319–325, 2001

Nigg JT, Goldsmith HH: Genetics of personality disorders: perspectives from personality and psychopathology research. Psychol Bull 115:346–380, 1994

Nilsson A: Lithium therapy and suicide risk. J Clin Psychiatry 60:85–88, 1999

Nurnberg HG, Martin GA, Pollack S: An empirical method to refine personality disorder classification using stepwise logistic regression modeling to develop diagnostic criteria and thresholds. Compr Psychiatry 35:409–419, 1994

Offer D, Offer J: Three developmental routes through normal male adolescence. Adolesc Psychiatry 4:121–141, 1975

Offer D, Kaiz M, Howard KI, et al: The altering of reported experiences. J Am Acad Child Adolesc Psychiatry 39:735–742, 2000

Ogawa K, Miya M, Watari A, et al: A long-term follow-up study of schizophrenia in Japan. Schizophr Bull 10:160–203, 1987

Ohberg A, Vuori E, Klaukka T, et al: Antidepressants and suicide mortality. J Affect Disord 50:225–233, 1998

Oldham JM: Development of the American Psychiatric Association practice guideline for the treatment of borderline personality disorder. J Personal Disord 16:109–112, 2002

Oldham JM, Skodol AE, Kellman D, et al: Diagnosis of DSM-III-R personality disorders by two structured interviews: patterns of comorbidity. Am J Psychiatry 149:213–220, 1992

Olds D, Henderson CR, Cole R, et al: Long-term effects of nurse home visitation on children's criminal and antisocial behavior. JAMA 280:1238–1244, 1998

O'Leary KM: Borderline personality disorder: neuropsychological testing results. Psychiatr Clin North Am 23:41–60, 2000

Packman WL, Harris EA: Legal issues and risk management in suicidal patients, in Risk Management with Suicidal Patients. Edited by Bongar B, Berman AL, Maris RW, et al. New York, Guilford, 1998, pp 150–186

Palmer BW, McClure FS, Jeste DV: Schizophrenia in late life: findings challenge traditional concepts. Harv Rev Psychiatry 9:51–58, 2001

Paris J: Intellectuality and emotionality in psychiatric residents. Can J Psychiatry 26:159–161, 1981

Paris J: Borderline Personality Disorder: a multidimensional approach. Washington, DC, American Psychiatric Press, 1994

Paris J: Memories of abuse in BPD: true or false? Harv Rev Psychiatry 3:10–17, 1995

Paris J: Social Factors in the Personality Disorders. New York, Cambridge University Press, 1996

Paris J: Antisocial and borderline personality disorders: two separate diagnoses or two aspects of the same psychopathology? Compr Psychiatry 38:237–242, 1997

Paris J: Anxious traits, anxious attachment, and anxious cluster personality disorders. Harv Rev Psychiatry 6:142–148, 1998a

Paris J: Working With Traits. Northvale, NJ, Jason Aronson, 1998b

Paris J: Nature and Nurture in Psychiatry: A Predisposition–Stress Model of Mental Disorders. Washington, DC, American Psychiatric Press, 1999

Paris J: Childhood precursors of borderline personality disorder. Psychiatr Clin North Am 23:77–88, 2000a

Paris J: The classification of personality disorders should be rooted in biology. J Personal Disord 14:127–136, 2000b

Paris J: Myths of Childhood. Philadelphia, PA, Brunner/Mazel, 2000c

Paris J: Chronic suicidality in borderline personality disorder. Psychiatr Serv 53:738–742, 2002a

Paris J: Implications of long-term outcome research for the management of patients with borderline personality disorder. Harv Rev Psychiatry 10:315–323, 2002b

Paris J, Braverman S: Successful and unsuccessful marriages in borderline patients. J Am Acad Psychoanal 23:153–166, 1995

Paris J, Zweig-Frank H: A 27-year follow-up of borderline patients. Compr Psychiatry 42:482–487, 2001

Paris J, Brown R, Nowlis D: Long-term follow-up of borderline patients in a general hospital. Compr Psychiatry 28:530–535, 1987

Paris J, Nowlis D, Brown R: Developmental factors in the outcome of borderline personality disorder. Compr Psychiatry 29:147–115, 1988

Paris J, Nowlis D, Brown R: Predictors of suicide in borderline personality disorder. Can J Psychiatry 34:8–9, 1989

Paris J, Zweig-Frank H, Guzder J: Psychological risk factors for borderline personality disorder in female patients. Compr Psychiatry 35:301–305, 1994a

Paris J, Zweig-Frank H, Guzder J: Risk factors for borderline personality in male outpatients. J Nerv Ment Dis 182:375–380, 1994b

Paris J, Zweig-Frank H, Guzder J: Psychological factors associated with homosexuality in males with borderline personality disorder. J Personal Disord 9:56–61, 1995

Paris J, Zelkowitz P, Guzder J, et al: Neuropsychological factors associated with borderline pathology in children. J Am Acad Child Adolesc Psychiatry 38:770–774, 1999

Parker G: Parental Overprotection: A Risk Factor in Psychosocial Development. New York, Grune and Stratton, 1983

Patterson GR, Yoerger K: A developmental model for late-onset delinquency. (Nebraska Symposium on Motivation; series editor Osgood DW) Motivation and Delinquency 44:119–177, 1997

Pepper CM, Klein DN, Anderson RL, et al: DSM-III-R Axis II comorbidity in dysthymia and major depression. Am J Psychiatry 152:239–247, 1995

Perry JC, Banon E, Ianni F: Effectiveness of psychotherapy for personality disorders. Am J Psychiatry 156:1312–1321, 1999

Petti TA, Vela RM: Borderline disorders of childhood: an overview. J Am Acad Child Adolesc Psychiatry 29:327–337, 1990

Pfohl B, Coryell W, Zimmerman M, Stangl D: DSM-III personality disorders: diagnostic overlap and internal consistency of individual DSM-III criteria. Compr Psychiatry 27:21–34, 1986

Pine F: On the concept of "borderline" in children. Psychoanal Study Child 29:341–368, 1974

Pinto A, Grapentine WL, Francis G, et al: Borderline personality disorder in adolescents: affective and cognitive features. J Am Acad Child Adolesc Psychiatry 35:1338–1343, 1996

Piper WE, Rosie JS, Joyce AS: Time-Limited Day Treatment for Personality Disorders: Integration of Research and Practice in a Group Program. Washington, DC, American Psychological Association, 1996

Plakun EM: Empirical studies on narcissism, in Psychiatric Treatment: Advances in Outcome Research. Edited by Mirin SM, Gosssett JT, Grob MC. Washington, DC, American Psychiatric Press, 1991, pp 195–212

Plakun EM, Burkhardt PE, Muller JP: 14-year follow-up of borderline and schizotypal personality disorders. Compr Psychiatry 27:448–455, 1985

Plomin R, Chuiper HM, Loehlin JC: Behavior genetics and personality, in Handbook of Personality Theory & Research. Edited by Pervin LA. New York, Guilford, 1990, pp 226–240

Plomin R, DeFries JC, McClearn GE, et al: Behavioral Genetics: A Primer, 3rd Edition. New York, W.H. Freeman, 2000

Pokorny AD: Prediction of suicide in psychiatric patients: report of a prospective study. Arch Gen Psychiatry 40:249–257, 1983

Pope HG, Jonas JM, Hudson JI: The validity of DSM-III borderline personality disorder. Arch Gen Psychiatry 40:23–30, 1983

Quartz S; Sejnowski T: The neural basis of cognitive development: a constructivist manifesto. Behav Brain Sci 20:537–596, 1997

Raine A, Lencz T, Bihrle S, et al: Reduced prefrontal gray matter volume and reduced autonomic activity in antisocial personality disorder. Arch Gen Psychiatry 57:119–127, 2001

Reich J, Yates W, Nduaguba M: Prevalence of DSM-III personality disorders in the community. Soc Psychiatry Psychiatr Epidemiol 24:12–16, 1989

Reiss D, Hetherington EM, Plomin R: The Relationship Code. Cambridge, MA, Harvard University Press, 2000

Rey JM, Singh M, Morris-Yates A, et al: Referred adolescents as young adults: the relationship between psychosocial functioning and personality disorder. Aust N Z J Psychiatry 31:219–226, 1997

Rich CL, Fowler RC, Fogarty LA, et al: San Diego suicide study: relationships between diagnoses and stressors. Arch Gen Psychiatry 45:589–594, 1988

Ricks DF, Berry JC: Family and symptom patterns that precede schizophrenia, in Life History Research in Psychopathology. Edited by Roff M, Ricks DF. Minneapolis, MN, University of Minnesota Press, 1970, pp 31–50

Rihmer Z, Rutz W, Pihlgren H: Depression and suicide on Gotland. An intensive study of all suicides before and after a depression-training programme for general practitioners. J Affect Disord 35:147–152, 1995

Rind B, Tromovitch P: A meta-analytic review of findings from national samples on psychological correlates of child sexual abuse. J Sex Res 34:237–255, 1997

Rind B, Tromovitch P, Bauserman R: A meta-analytic examination of assumed properties of child sexual abuse using college samples. Psychol Bull 124:22–53, 1998

Rinne T, van den Brink W, Worters L, et al: SSRI treatment of borderline personality disorder. Am J Psychiatry 159:2048–2054, 2002

Riso LP, Klein DN, Ferro T, et al: Understanding the comorbidity between early onset dysthymia and cluster B personality disorders: a family study. Am J Psychiatry 153:900–906, 1996

Riso LP, Klein DN, Anderson RL, et al: A family study of outpatients with borderline personality disorder and no history of mood disorder. J Personal Disord 14:208–217, 2000

Robins E, Guze SB: Establishment of diagnostic validity in psychiatric illness: its application to schizophrenia. Am J Psychiatry 126:107–111, 1970

Robins LN: Deviant Children Grown Up. Baltimore, MD, Williams & Wilkins, 1966

Robins LN: Sturdy childhood predictors of adult outcome. Psychol Med 8:611–622, 1978

Robins LN, Regier DA (eds): Psychiatric Disorders in America. New York, Free Press, 1991

Robson KR: The Borderline Child. New York, McGraw Hill, 1983

Ronningstam EF: Narcissistic personality disorder and pathological narcissism: long-term stability and presence in Axis I disorders, in Disorders of Narcissism. Edited by Ronningstam EF. Washington, DC, American Psychiatric Press, 1998, pp 375–414

Rosenthal D: The Genain Quadruplets. New York, Basic Books, 1968

Rothbart MK, Ahadi SA, Evans DE: Temperament and personality: origins and outcomes. J Pers Soc Psychol 78:122–135, 2000

Rutter M: Psychosocial resilience and protective mechanisms. Am J Orthopsychiatry 57:316–331, 1987a

Rutter M: Temperament, Personality, and Personality Development, Br J Psychiatry 150:443–448, 1987b

Rutter M: Pathways from childhood to adult life. J Child Psychol Psychiatry 30:23–51, 1989

Rutter M: Nature, nurture, and psychopathology: a new look at an old topic. Dev Psychopathol 3:125–136, 1991

Rutter M, Maughan B: Psychosocial adversities in psychopathology. J Personal Disord 11:4–18, 1997

Rutter M, Quinton D: Parental psychiatric disorder: effects on children. Psychol Med 14:853–880, 1984

Rutter M, Rutter M: Developing Minds: Challenge and Continuity Across the Life Span. New York, Basic Books, 1993

Rutter M, Smith DJ: Psychosocial Disturbances in Young People. Cambridge, UK, Cambridge University Press, 1995

Rutz W: Preventing suicide and premature death by education and treatment. J Affect Disord 62:123–129, 2001

Sabo AN, Gunderson JG, Najavits LM, et al: Changes in self-destructiveness of borderline patients in psychotherapy: a prospective follow up. J Nerv Ment Dis 183:370–376, 1995

Sackett DL, Richardson WS, Rosenberg W, et al: Evidence-Based Medicine. Edinburgh, Scotland, Churchill Livingstone, 1997

Salzman JP, Salzman C, Wolfson AN, et al: Association between borderline personality structure and history of childhood abuse in adult volunteers. Compr Psychiatry 34:254–257, 1993

Salzman C, Wolfson AN, Schatzberg A, et al: Effect of fluoxetine on anger in symptomatic volunteers with borderline personality disorder. J Clin Psychopharmacol 15:23–29, 1995

Samuels J, Eaton WW, Bienvenu J, et al: Prevalence and correlates of personality disorders in a community sample. Br J Psychiatry 180:536–542, 2002

Sanderson C, Swenson C, Bohus M: A critique of the American Psychiatric Association practice guideline for the treatment of patients with borderline personality disorder. J Personal Disord 16:122–129, 2002

Sato T, Takeichi M: Lifetime prevalence of specific psychiatric disorders in a general medicine clinic. Gen Hosp Psychiatry 15:224–233, 1993

Schacter DL: Searching for Memory. New York, Basic Books, 1996

Scheel KR: The empirical basis of dialectical behavior therapy: summary, critique, and implications. Clin Psychol Sci Pract 7:68–86, 2000

Schmideberg M: The borderline patient, in The American Handbook of Psychiatry, Vol I. Edited by Arieti S. New York, Basic Books, 1959, pp 398–416

Schneidman ES: Psychotherapy with suicidal patients. Suicide and Life-Threatening Behavior 11:341–348, 1981

Schuckit MA, Smith TL: An 8-year follow-up of 450 sons of alcoholic and control subjects. Arch Gen Psychiatry 53:202–210, 1996

Seivewright H, Tyrer P, Johnson T: Prediction of outcome in neurotic disorder: a 5-year prospective study. Psychol Med 28:1149–1157, 1998

Seivewright H, Tyrer P, Johnson T: Change in personality status in neurotic disorders. Lancet 359:2253–2254, 2002

Shea MT, Pilkonis PA, Beckham E, et al: Personality disorders and treatment outcome in the NIMH Treatment of Depression Collaborative Research Program. Am J Psychiatry 147:711–718, 1990

Shea MT, Elkin I, Imber SD, et al: Course of depressive symptoms over follow-up: findings from the National Institute of Mental Health Treatment of Depression Collaborative Research Program. Arch Gen Psychiatry 49:782–787, 1992

Shulman KI, Tohen M, Satlin A, et al: Mania compared with unipolar depression in old age. Am J Psychiatry 149:341–345, 1992

Siever LJ, Davis KL: A psychobiological perspective on the personality disorders. Am J Psychiatry 148:1647–1658, 1991

Siever LJ, Kalus OF, Keefe RS: The boundaries of schizophrenia. Psych Clin North Am 162:17–44, 1993

Siever LJ, New AS, Kirrane R, et al: New biological research strategies for personality disorders, in Biology of Personality Disorders. Edited by Silk KR. Washington, DC, American Psychiatric Press, 1998, pp 27–62

Silver D: Psychotherapy of the characterologically difficult patient. Can J Psychiatry 28:513–521, 1983

Silver D, Cardish R: BPD outcome studies: psychotherapy implications. Paper presented to the American Psychiatric Association, New Orleans, LA, May 1991

Skodol AE, Buckley P, Charles E: Is there a characteristic pattern in the treatment history of clinic outpatients with borderline personality? J Nerv Ment Dis 171:405–410, 1983

Skodol AE, Gunderson JG, McGlashan TH, et al: Functional impairment in patients with schizotypal, borderline, avoidant, or obsessive-compulsive personality disorder. Am J Psychiatry 159:276–283, 2002

Skoog I: Detection of preclinical Alzheimer's disease. N Engl J Med 343:502–503, 2000

Small GW, Mazziota JC, Collins MT: Apoliprotein E type 4 allele and cerebral glucose metabolism in relatives at risk for familial Alzheimer disease. JAMA 273:942–947, 1995

Snarey JR, Vaillant GE: How lower- and working-class youth become middle-class adults: the association between ego defense mechanisms and upward social mobility. Child Dev 56:899–910, 1985

Sobin C, Blundell ML, Conry A, et al: Early, non-psychotic deviant behavior in schizophrenia: a possible endophenotypic marker for genetic studies. Psychiatry Res 101:101–113, 2001

Soldz S, Vaillant GE: The Big Five personality traits and the life course: a 45-year longitudinal study. J Res Personal 33:208–232, 1999

Soloff P: Psychopharmacological treatment of borderline personality disorder. Psychiatr Clin North Am 23:169–192, 2000

Soloff PH, Millward JW: Developmental histories of borderline patients. Compr Psychiatry 23:574–588, 1983

Soloff PH, Cornelius J, George A, et al: Efficacy of phenelzine and haloperidol in borderline personality disorder. Arch Gen Psychiatry 50:377–385, 1993

Statistics Canada. Health Reports. Supplement No. 13.2: #2. Ottawa, Canada, 1990

Steiger H, Zanko M: Sexual trauma among eating-disordered, psychiatric, and normal female groups. J Interpers Violence 5:74–86, 1990

Stein DJ, Hollander E, Cohen L, et al: Neuropsychiatric impairment in impulsive personality disorders. Psychiatry Res 48:257–266, 1993

Stern A: Psychoanalytic investigation of and therapy in the borderline group of neuroses. Psychoanal Q 7:467–489, 1938

Stevenson J, Goodman R: Association between behaviour at age 3 years and adult criminality. Br J Psychiatry 179:197–202, 2001

Stevenson J, Meares R: An outcome study of psychotherapy for patients with borderline personality disorder. Am J Psychiatry 149:358–362, 1992

Stone MH: The Fate of Borderline Patients. New York, Guilford, 1990

Stravynski A, Belisle M, Macouiller M, et al: The treatment of avoidant personality disorder by social skills training in the clinic or in real-life settings. Can J Psychiatry 39:377–383, 1994

Sudak HS, Ford AB, Rushforth NB: Suicide in the Young. Boston, MA, John Wright, 1984

Sullivan PF, Neale MC, Kendler KS: Genetic epidemiology of major depression: review and metanalysis. Am J Psychiatry 157:1552–1562, 2000

Sutker PB, Bugg F, West JA: Antisocial personality disorder, in Comprehensive Handbook of Psychopathology, 2nd Edition. Edited by Sutker PB, Adams HE. New York, Kluwer, 1993, pp 337–369

Svrakic DM, Whitehead C, Przybeck TR, et al: Differential diagnosis of personality disorders by the seven-factor model of temperament and character. Arch Gen Psychiatry 50:991–999, 1993

Swartz M, Blazer D, George L, et al: Estimating the prevalence of borderline personality disorder in the community. J Personal Disord 4:257–272, 1990

Szmukler G, Dare C, Treasure J (eds): Handbook of Eating Disorders: Theory, Treatment and Research. Chichester, UK, John Wiley, 1995

Tiet QQ, Wasserman GA, Loeber R, et al: Developmental and sex differences in types of conduct problems. J Child Family Studies 10:181–197, 2001

Tohen M, Bromet E, Murphy JM, et al: Psychiatric epidemiology. Harv Rev Psychiatry 8:111–125, 2000

Tooby J, Cosmides L: The psychological foundations of culture, in The Adapted Mind: Evolutionary Psychology and the Generation of Culture. Edited by Barkow JH, Cosmides L, Tooby J. New York, Oxford University Press, 1992, pp 19–136

Torgersen S: Correlates of Personality Disorder Diagnoses. Paper presented to the International Society for the Study of Personality Disorders, Dublin, Ireland, June 1995

Torgersen S, Lygren S, Oien PA, et al: A twin study of personality disorders. Compr Psychiatry 41:416–425, 2000

Torgersen S, Kringlen E, Cramer V: The prevalence of personality disorders in a community sample. Arch Gen Psychiatry 58:590–596, 2001

Tremblay RE, Pihl RO, Vitaro F, et al: Predicting early onset of male antisocial behavior from preschool behavior. Arch Gen Psychiatry 51:732–739, 1994

Trivedi MH, Kleiber BA: Using treatment algorithms for the effective management of treatment-resistant depression. J Clin Psychiatry 62(suppl):25–29, 2001

Tyrer P: Practice guideline for the treatment of borderline personality disorder: a bridge too far. J Personal Disord 16:113–118, 2002

Tyrer P, Seivewright H: Outcome of Personality Disorders, in Personality Disorders: Diagnosis, Management, and Course, 2nd Edition. Edited by Tyrer P. Oxford, UK, Butterworth Heinemann, 2000, pp 105–125

Vaglum P, Friis S, Karterud S, et al: Stability of the severe personality disorder diagnosis: a 2- to 5-year prospective study. J Personal Disord 10:348–353, 1996

Vaillant GE: Adaptation to Life. Cambridge, MA, Little Brown, 1977

Vaillant GE: Is there a natural history of addiction? J Nerv Ment Dis 70:41–57, 1992

Vaillant GE: The Natural History of Alcoholism Revisited. Cambridge, MA, Harvard University Press, 1995

Vaillant GE, Mukamal K: Successful aging. Am J Psychiatry 158:839–847, 2001

Verheul R, ven den Bosch LMC, Maarten WJ, et al: Dialectical behaviour therapy for women with borderline personality disorder: 12-month, randomised clinical trial in The Netherlands. Br J Psychiatry 182:135–140, 2003

Vitaro F, Tremblay RE: Impact of a prevention program on aggressive children's friendships and social adjustment. J Abnorm Child Psychol 224:57–75, 1994

Vito E, Ladame F, Orlandini A: Adolescence and personality disorders: current perspectives on a controversial problem, in Treatment of Personality Disorders. Edited by Derksen J, Maffei C. New York, Kluwer Academic/Plenum, 1999, pp 77–95

Waldinger RJ, Gunderson JG: Completed psychotherapies with borderline patients. Am J Psychother 38:190–201, 1984

Walker EF, Savoie T, Davis D: Neuromotor precursors of schizophrenia. Schizophr Bull 20:441–451, 1994

Wallerstein R: Forty-Two Lives in Treatment. New York, Guilford, 1986

Weckerly J: Pediatric bipolar mood disorder. J Dev Behav Pediatr 23:42–56, 2002

Weinberg MK, Tronick EZ, Cohn JF, et al: Gender differences in emotional expressivity and self-regulation during early infancy. Dev Psychol 35:175–188, 1999

Weinberger DR: Implications of normal brain development for the pathogenesis of schizophrenia. Arch Gen Psychiatry 44:660–669, 1987

Weiss G, Hechtman L: Hyperactive Children Grown Up, 2nd Edition. New York, Guilford, 1993

Weiss M, Zelkowitz P, Feldman R, et al: Psychopathology in offspring of mothers with borderline personality disorder. Can J Psychiatry 41:285–290, 1996

Weissman MM: The epidemiology of personality disorders: a 1990 update. J Personal Disord 7(suppl):44–62, 1993

Weissman MM, Klerman GL: Gender and depression. Trends Neurosci 8:416–420, 1985

Weissman MM, Bland RC, Canino GJ, et al: Cross-national epidemiology of major depressive and bipolar disorder. JAMA 276:298–299, 1996

Weissman MM, Greenwald S, Wickramaratne P, et al: What happens to depressed men? Application of the Stirling County criteria. Harv Rev Psychiatry 5:1–6, 1997

Weissman MM, Wolk S, Goldstein RB, et al: Depressed adolescents grown up. JAMA 281:1707–1713, 1999

Werble B: Second follow-up study of borderline patients. Arch Gen Psychiatry 23:3–7, 1970

Werner EE, Smith RS: Overcoming the Odds: High Risk Children from Birth to Adulthood. New York, Cornell University Press, 1992

West DJ, Farrington DP: Who Becomes Delinquent? London, Heinemann, 1973

Westen D, Chang C: Personality pathology in adolescence: a review, in Adolescent Psychiatry: Developmental and Clinical Studies. Edited by Esman A, Flaherty LT. Hillsdale, NJ, Analytic Press, 25:61–100, 2000

Widom CS: Posttraumatic stress disorder in abused and neglected children grown up. Am J Psychiatry 156:1223–1229, 1999

Wilkinson DG: The suicide rate in schizophrenia. Br J Psychiatry 140:138–141, 1982

Williams L: A "classic" case of borderline personality disorder. Psychiatr Serv 49:173–174, 1998

Winokur G, Tsuang M: The Natural History of Mania, Depression, and Schizophrenia. Washington, DC, American Psychiatric Press, 1996

Winston A, Laikin M, Pollack J, et al: Short-term psychotherapy of personality disorders. Am J Psychiatry 151:190–194, 1994

Wolberg AR: The Borderline Patient. New York, Intercontinental Medical, 1973

Wolff S, Townshend R, McGuire RJ, et al: 'Schizoid' personality in childhood and adult life, II: adult adjustment and the continuity with schizotypal personality disorder. Br J Psychiatry 159:620–629, 1991

Woody GE, McLennan T, Luborsky L, et al: Sociopathy and psychotherapy outcome. Arch Gen Psychiatry 42:1081–1086, 1985

Wu P, Hoven CW, Cohen P, et al: Factors associated with use of mental health services for depression by children and adolescents. Psychiatr Serv 52:189–195, 2001

Wulsin LR, Vaillant GE, Wells VE: A systematic review of the mortality of depression. Psychosom Med 61:6–17, 1999

Yochelson S, Samenow S: The Criminal Personality. New York, Jason Aronson, 1976

Young JE: Cognitive Therapy for Personality Disorders: A Schema-Focused Approach, 3rd Edition. Sarasota, FL, Professional Resource Press, 1999

Zahn-Waxler C, Klimes-Dougam B, Slattery MJ: Internalizing problems of childhood and adolescence: prospects, pitfalls, and progress in understanding the development of anxiety and depression. Dev Psychopathol 12:443–466, 2000

Zanarini MC: Borderline personality as an impulse spectrum disorder, in Borderline Personality Disorder: Etiology and Treatment. Edited by Paris J. Washington, DC, American Psychiatric Press, 1993, pp 67–86

Zanarini MC: Childhood experiences associated with the development of borderline personality disorder. Psychiatr Clin North Am 23:89–101, 2000

Zanarini MC, Frankenburg FR: Emotional hypochondriasis, hyperbole, and the borderline patient. J Psychother Pract Res 3:25–36, 1994

Zanarini MC, Frankenburg FR: Olanzapine treatment of female borderline personality disorder patients: a double-blind, placebo-controlled pilot study. J Clin Psychiatry 62:849–854, 2001

Zanarini MC, Gunderson JG, Frankenburg FR: The revised diagnostic interview for borderlines: discriminating BPD from other Axis II disorders. J Personal Disord 3:10–18, 1989

Zanarini MC, Gunderson JG, Frankenburg FR: Cognitive features of borderline personality disorder. Am J Psychiatry 147:57–63, 1990

Zanarini MC, Frankenburg FR, Dubo ED, et al: Axis II comorbidity of borderline personality disorder. Compr Psychiatry 39:296–302, 1998

Zanarini MC, Frankenburg FR, Khera GS, et al: Treatment histories of borderline inpatients. Compr Psychiatry 42:144–150, 2001

Zanarini MC, Frankenburg FR, Hennen J, et al: The longitudinal course of borderling psychopathology: 6-year prospective follow-up of the phenomenology of borderline personality disorder. Am J Psychiatry 160:274–283, 2003

Zeitlin D: The Natural History of Psychiatric Disorders in Children. Oxford, Oxford University Press, 1986

Zelkowitz P, Guzder J, Paris J: Diatheses and stressors in borderline pathology of childhood: the role of neuropsychological risk and trauma, J Am Acad Child Adolesc Psychiatry 40:100–105, 2001

Zoccolillo M, Pickles A, Quinton D, et al: The outcome of childhood conduct disorder: implications for defining adult personality disorder and conduct disorder. Psychol Med 22:971–986, 1992

Zoccolillo M, Tremblay R, Vitaro F: DSM-III and DSM-III-R criteria for conduct disorder in preadolescent girls: specific but insensitive. J Am Acad Child Adolesc Psychiatry 35:461–470, 1996

Zubenko GS, George AW, Soloff PH, et al: Sexual practices among patients with borderline personality disorder. Am J Psychiatry 144:748–752, 1987

Zweig-Frank H, Paris J: Recollections of emotional neglect and overprotection in borderline patients. Am J Psychiatry 148:648–651, 1991

Zweig-Frank H, Paris J: The five factor model of personality in borderline personality disorder. Can J Psychiatry 40:523–526, 1995

Zweig-Frank H, Paris J: Predictors of outcomes in a 27 year follow-up of patients with borderline personality disorder. Compr Psychiatry 43:103–107, 2002

Index

*Page numbers printed in **boldface** type refer to tables or figures.*